HOLISTIC

EXORCISM

Manual compiled by *John Living*
Retired Professional Engineer, Spiritual Healer

The world we see is small in comparison to the world we do not see.   By writing this very interesting book, John Living gives us a look at the unseen world.

Raymon Grace

John Living

HOLISTIC EXORCISM

Published by The Holistic Intuition Society

Our Website: www.in2it.ca

Toll Free Canada & USA: 1-866-369-7464

For other books by John Living see:

www.in2it.ca/Books.htm

Holistic Exorcism
Index of Contents

About the Author

About the Author

John Living was one of the first intake of the Royal Military Academy Sandhurst to be commissioned by HM Queen Elizabeth II - in 1952. He was taught to Dowse as a young officer in the Corps of Royal Engineers.

After attending university, John left the army and started business in real estate, and was elected as a member of the County Borough Council of Southend-on-Sea.

In 1965 he went to Jamaica, becoming the Resident Engineer of a major road, dyke, and bridge construction project. He later joined the National Water Authority of Jamaica, becoming the executive assistant to the General Manager. In 1976 John emigrated to Canada.

Now retired, John has been a Royal Engineer, a member of the Engineering Institute of Jamaica, a Chartered Civil Engineer, and a Professional Engineer. His main interest now is Dowsing and Healing, including Exorcism.

John was a co-founder of the Holistic Intuition Society to organize Dowsing in the Canadian Prairie Provinces - the society membership is now part of the Canadian Society of Questers, of which he is an Honorary Life member.

His articles have been published in the journals of the American, Australian, British, Canadian, New Zealand, and Swedish Dowsing societies.

John taught many people to Dowse (which he calls 'Intuition Technology') and has written a number of books on Dowsing, Healing, and Exorcism.

He now lives in a cabin overlooking the golf course on Galiano Island, halfway between Vancouver and Victoria in British Columbia. Apart from writing books and exorcising unwanted spirit attachments, John's main employment is as a butler to Pedro, a member of the famous Labrador and Husky families.

In his 'spare time' he acts like Sherlock Holmes (even smoking a Peterson pipe) to discover the intricacies of life, which he compares to a multi-dimensional jig-saw puzzle.

Chapter 1

Overview

I trust that it will be of great assistance to you in helping people to be free of the various forms of interference from various dimensions, including remnants of loved ones who have passed on and those often called Demonic or Spirit Possession.

The comments that I make are the result of asking the higher levels of Spirit for guidance - especially about aspects of the Spirit domains about which we all know very little. To do this, I ask questions such as "If I knew how xxx works, what would the correct answer be?" where xxx indicates the actual information that I need. I then 'hear' the needed answer.

Most people do not understand that there are many levels in the non-physical dimensions. Some explanations may seem to vary - but all these may be correct, just as understood by different people from varying aspects and subject to their individual interpretations.

Fragments and Possession

What is meant by 'possession'? It is the interference by others (physical and non-physical) in the mental, emotional, spiritual, or physical well-being of a person. Exorcism is the process of removing such interference; other healing modalities may be needed to overcome the residual effects of such possession.

We are all elements of Spirit having experience in the physical plane. Our own Spirit comes to our being as its consciousness, and usually diversifies to handle different aspects of our life. If there is trauma, such a diversified part may detach from our consciousness and have a separate existence as a fragment - but usually trying to keep close to the main consciousness.

In this way the various diversified parts activate our life by guiding us to do different tasks at various times - this being accomplished by taking control and operating our brain neurons (and hence our speech and other actions) as so needed.

Fragments from others (especially those released at the major trauma of death) may attach to us if attracted for whatever reason - our thoughts being a major attraction, since the non-physical domains are primarily domains of thought.

My understanding is that the Heavens above the Astral are domains of thought; that the Astral Heavens (to which humans aspire to return) are domains of thought forms; that the physical planes of matter could be considered as comprised of condensed thought forms; and that in all cases the higher levels have great influence over the lower levels.

In this context consider the Astral plane of the earth to be separate from the Astral Heavens; if a Soul is 'earthbound' it is active in the Astral plane of the earth and has not reached the Astral Heavens. This is also the case with fragments that have detached from the Spirit Consciousness.

These fragments then attach to people who are alive, and are the most common sources of unwanted and negative influences upon human beings.

In his book 'Healing Lost Souls', William Baldwin writes: *"Attached entities seldom make their presence known to the host; spirit attachment is usually a surprise to the client. Although the condition of spirit interference is nearly universal, most people are not aware of these parasitic attachments."*

The diseases from which the person suffered (and may have caused their death) may manifest from the fragment into you; these cause many illnesses that the medical systems fail to heal! Changes in character often occur, causing problems in your social and business life.

Your likes and dislikes change. Exorcism is needed!

Healing such as by exorcism is best done at a distance - by an experienced exorcist.

Types of Possession

In using the term 'Possession' we include also the negative influences originating from those who are still alive in the physical plane of existence - their hateful thoughts, curses, and hexes.

Most common are the attachments of Souls (or their fragments) from deceased relatives - including the Souls of children who were not born or died young, and the earthbound parts of family members (and close friends) who have not ascended in the correct manner and seek to continue their earthly existence by invading relatives still alive, especially young children.

Such fragments will often hide in the muscles of the victim; the more developed will also move around within the muscle system - usually the medical professions find that their medicines are not effective in healing the pains. They say "it is all your imagination!"

Worse possession, however, comes from the invasion of deceased addicts when protection is low from drugs or alcohol; and by earthbound Souls (or those who have lost their way) when the subject is unconscious - due to an accident, or especially when under anaesthetics in a hospital.

Even the best of intent from a deceased family member (such as a parent meaning to help a child) can have most unfortunate side effects. Very often the subject then suffers from illnesses brought in to their own body by the deceased relative - sometimes immediately, or perhaps at the age when the 'donor' died!

The worst of all is when a person is attacked by a 'Real Nasty', as described by Dr José Lacerda de Azevedo, M.D., of Brazil in his book 'Spirit and Matter'. He describes the way that those who call on the help of the dark forces find themselves bound to obey the darkness after death, how they are incarcerated in dungeons, and how they are sent on missions to hurt people - and severely punished if not successful. This is outlined in Chapters 3 and 4.

Exorcism

Most people involved in exorcism have little or no knowledge of the darkest side of existence - and are unable to help those who are attacked.

Our Spiritual friends with whom we work have carefully explored these domains, and found ways to release those incarcerated and heal them to prevent further subjection by the dark forces.

All these possessing spirit entities may also carry attachments or be possessed by other unwanted spirit entities (a 'piggy-back' effect) since when a person dies these often remain with them.

Dealing with such situations is fraught with difficulties. In many instances when such a possessing spirit entity is removed it can attach itself to the person doing the removal - with terrible consequences when a 'real nasty' is involved.

Another factor is that when you are working to help someone who is close to you healing (including exorcism) often fails due to the interference from your emotions, beliefs, and feelings.

So it is preferable for all work to remove possessing entities (of all descriptions) to be done by those who are very experienced in the work of exorcism - who take the needed personal precautions and who ensure that the entities removed are correctly healed and taken to their rightful place.

Experienced exorcists have had great success with the exorcism of 'real nasties' at a distance (even at 4,000 miles) using the method detailed in this book. Our attitude is that there is no charge for the exorcism itself, but a charge is made for the time and expenses that are expended in the work.

Additional healing is given to clear the aura of negativity and to work with the Heart and sub-conscious of the subject - to remove problems resulting from (and sometimes causing) such possession.

Typical Symptoms of Possession

Include a lack of energy, weakness in the body, severe depression, disturbed thoughts, and/or irrational thinking. In general a person who is possessed can be identified as being extremely negative and severely depressed, - and especially if anti-social behaviour is exhibited.

Indications of possession include:
Strong negativity
Deep depression
Rapid mood changes
Uncontrolled temper
Self inflicted harm

Even one or two of these indicators may be a signal of possession.

We have also found a number of cases where deceased church members have invaded a person who has abandoned their religion, so as to try to force them to return to their old beliefs - this is most prevalent by evangelistic relatives!

Observations by Parapsychologists

George Meek writes in his book 'After we Die, What Then?':

"Those departing souls who arrive on the lowest of the astral planes find they lack physical bodies and are bewildered ... Some may be attracted by the energy field ... of nearby mortals ... who may be friends or relatives attending the funeral ... attaching to the auras of those still in the flesh.

They will influence the possessed person with their own thoughts, impart their own emotions, and weaken his/her will power. In some cases this takeover can be so complete that they will actually control the possessed person's actions, often producing great distress, harmful mental disturbances, and suffering."

From 'Body, Mind, and Spirit' by Dr Peter Albright:

"Who or what are these entities, and where do they come from? In our culture persons are not very well educated about or prepared for death, as Elizabeth Kubler-Ross has found. ... You get what you expect, and find that death leaves them still functioning as personalities but without an 'earth suit' to wear. They think that they cannot function without one, so seek entrance to any 'earth suit' that is handy and still operating which may be open to them.

The results for the host can be confusing, to say the least. Since the invasion affects primarily the sub-conscious mind, the host may have little or no awareness of what is going on. Even if the host is aware of new problems and difficulties, he will not be aware of the cause."

A personal comment by John Living:

My grandfather died at age 93 when I was 9 years old. He always smoked a cigar each day. When I tried to stop smoking, I found (using Gary Craig's Emotional Freedom Techniques - EFT) that my Grandfather was 'in me' and was 'encouraging' me to smoke!

This was also encouraged by an Indian 'helper' who was a most accomplished 'medicine man' and 'pipe carrier'.

Hypochondriac - Forever Ill

It is a common occurrence to take on the illness of a possessing spirit entity - hence the usual poor health of a person who is possessed; even a child will reflect poor health when a spirit entity becomes attached.

A person whose physical illness has been medically diagnosed as imaginary may well be the victim of possession! To further complicate the case a person may have several possessing spirit entities 'on board', each having different illnesses and symptoms.

As a result, the victim goes from doctor to doctor, usually getting diagnoses that conflict.

Baby Souls

When a baby is conceived but not born (or dies young) its Spirit Consciousness often fragments due to the trauma of death and attaches to the mother; if another baby is conceived it may then 'join' with the new baby soul - this may result in an extra strong male or female personality (if the souls are of the same sex) or to a lesbian/gay adult should the baby souls have different sexual orientations.

If the baby soul remains attached to the mother then the mother can expect problems in later life - and without any realization that a baby soul is involved.   For more information read 'A Cry from the Womb' by Gwendolyn Awen Jones (ISBN9780974073019) outlined in Chapter 5.

Personal Knowledge of Possessed Person

More accurate readings can be obtained when the exorcist knows little about the client. The exorcist must constantly guard himself from letting his rational mind influence the information that he receives.

For example, should the exorcist's rational mind decide that it is ridiculous for a certain person to be possessed, the sub-conscious will 'oblige', and the person will be given a clean 'bill of health' even though the truth may be otherwise.

This is of particular importance when we are dealing with someone who is 'close' to us, such as a friend or relative. Our rational mind will distort facts to accord with our personal feelings and emotions.

So it is best if the exorcist has only the details, such as name, age, and address - with any photo, etc, to ensure that the correct person is being contacted. Hair and/or a blood sample is also useful for this purpose - to ensure that an actual person is correctly identified.

It seems to be far more effective (and safer!) to do an exorcism at a distance (even thousands of miles away) than to be with the (possibly) possessed person.

Exorcism 'face to face' can result in the exorcist being attacked by the possessed person, and by the possessing spirit transferring to the exorcist.

More Information on Entities

The best books on the various planes of existence are those of Charles Leadbeater and of Annie Besant, from the Theosophical Society; 'Entity Possession' by Samuel Sagan M.D. of the Clairvision School in Australia gives excellent details of fragments and their effects. 'Healing Lost Souls' by William Baldwin gives a detailed description of cause and effect.

Soul Fragments

When a person dies then in most cases the Soul Spirit departs to the Heavens of the Astral Plane, minus any fragments. If a fragment is associated with 'stuff' from the person's etheric body, then it has an individual existence in the Astral plane of the Earth - but needs 'life force' to continue its existence; this it usually gets from attaching to a person who is still alive.

Each fragment can be considered to be a particular aspect of the person - having a precise task that was a characteristic (known or suppressed) of that person. Its thoughts are only how it can continue in its given task.

All these fragments 'float' in the Astral plane of the earth, seeking someone to whom they can attach - as 'Like seeks Like' they seek a person with whom they have a genetic, emotional, or mental similarity.

When attached to a person the fragment can by-pass the person's Spirit Consciousness and take over - then manipulate the neurons of the person's brain to carry out its designated task. This may include causing hurts, diseases, etc., associated with the trauma that caused it to become a fragment.

Some fragments persist for many hundreds of years. If anger or hate is involved, they will seek the vibrational pattern of the subject of such anger or hate - this explains some 'past life' experiences; however the past life may be that of another person having a similar vibrational pattern to that of the person to whom the fragment is attached.

When a person (especially a child) is subject to what it perceives as a major trauma then a piece of the Soul may fragment (usually keeping close to the Soul) but the trauma may permit a foreign soul fragment to attach to the Soul. Lonely children may invite 'playmates' (Lost Souls or fragments) who cause problems in later life.

Clairvoyants looking at fragments may see just a face, eyes, or only a mouth - another indication that what is there is not the real person, but only a fragment.

Inhabitants of the Astral Plane

In the Astral Plane (and higher planes) even thoughts have shapes - and are as real in that plane as is an item in the physical world. Hence a person's thoughts (good or bad) have an effect on the subject of such thoughts, no matter the distance involved.

It is also the way in which Human Beings can use their thoughts (with will power) to influence the inhabitants of the Astral Plane - such as sending them Healing and Love (including exorcism!)

Animal souls (including those of reptiles and birds - even of extinct species) can be seen by clairvoyants in the Astral Plane.

Hexes, Curses, and Negative Energies

Hexes and curses (including miasms from other ages) remain in place until cleared; this is why so many places have bad energies - a curse, etc. was placed many years ago, but never cleared, and so remains effective. Ghosts may manifest after a very traumatic death.

In a similar way a bad energy sent to a person may affect many future generations (curses from a past life may have the same effect on the soul) and need to be removed.

Sorcery may include giving instructions to inhabitants of the Astral Plane to cause harm to a subject. Poltergeist activity is often the result of Soul fragmentation or attachment.

It is probable that when a hex is placed a portion of the Spirit Consciousness of the hex-maker detaches as a fragment to implement the hex.

Spirit Possession

This is primarily when a Spirit entity that is not 'In the Light' has control over a person. An 'earth bound' soul (or fragment) may be in this category.

Sometimes this is accomplished by pretending to be an Angel or Spirit Guide, persuading the person to work with them, and so gaining entry - so beware if you have any doubts about your guides! Any sign of giving orders, or trying to cause harm to anyone, or giving any negative hints should be taken as a signal that they are not 'In the Light'.

The 'Light' is the light, radiation, field, etc. of Love - not the love of sex or possession, but 'Unconditional True Holy Love', best described as 'Namaste'.

A Note

This information is not meant to scare you - but to help you to realize that attachment and possession of various types is far more prevalent than is generally recognized (and is often ignored by the medical system, who treat the symptoms, usually not the cause!) - and to offer you a solution to problems which may otherwise fail to be effectively treated and so cause serious illnesses, major problems in life, and often an early death.

Forgiveness

It is most important that you successfully and completely forgive all who have ever caused you hurt or harm, forgiving from Soul and Spirit as well as mind.

This can be very difficult, especially in cases of abuse by family members. It is suggested that in such cases you accept that what was done occurred as a result of karma (or possession), and was not directly the fault of the perpetrators.

The key is to find some 'reason' to allow you to forgive, no matter how difficult this is for the rational mind. Failure to be so forgiving will prevent any exorcism from being effective - you may get short term relief, but problems will re-occur.

A detailed example of a forgiveness statement is attached at Appendix A.

Understanding 'The Matrix'

In 1944, Max Planck, the father of quantum theory, shocked the world by saying that this 'matrix" is where the birth of stars, the DNA of life, and everything between originates - a place where all things begin, the place of pure energy that simply 'is'. In this quantum incubator for reality, everything is possible.

The MATRIX provides:
- The container for the universe
- The bridge between your imagination and your reality
- The mirror in our world for what you create in your beliefs

This link in our understanding is missing in many people.

To tap the force of this matrix, we must understand how it works and speak the language that it recognizes - the secret of the Divine Matrix, as found in the coded language of our cherished traditions and verified in today's science.

The Matrix connects us as ONE. When we have a thought, it goes out to the Matrix, and then returns as our life experience.

We can change our lives by changing the thoughts or pictures in the Matrix.

This field or Matrix is all around us, and connects us to our past. We hold our traumas and stressful life experiences in the Matrix, where they can influence our every thought pattern, behaviour and action. These are held not just as memories but as specific energy bodies, which have been named 'Energy Conscious Holograms' - the ECHOs in Karl Dawson's 'Matrix Re-imprinting' work.

Sometimes we carry around pictures in our minds from the past, for years. At the time the event occurred, part of the self splits off and goes into the Matrix. It is a dissociated part, a fragment, that becomes an 'Energy Consciousness Hologram', or ECHO.

Our energy field is still vibrating in alignment with the negative picture or event, so we are 'stuck' in the old, painful memories and pictures that are in the Matrix. We also continue to attract more such negative experiences, because experience follows energy vibration.

Karl Dawson has developed a wonderful system to change these old, painful memories and pictures into becoming happy and beneficial - this aspect seems to be ignored by most systems that work with timelines.

Karl has written a book 'Matrix Reappointing using EFT' ISBN 9781848502499 published by Hay House and available on Amazon.

In his DVD series Karl tells how such a change has an effect not just on the person directly affected, but also on the others involved. This can be expected to be of great help to those now dead who were associated with the events.

Tales from the Masters

I do not pretend to 'know it all' - and so I have included extracts from other authors that I consider to be exceptional leaders in this field.

The extract from **Dr Baldwin's** paper in Chapter 2 is a wonderful introduction to the overall aspect of Spirit Possession - "investigators in this field estimate that between 70% and 100% of the population are affected or influenced by one or more discarnate spirit entities at some time in their life."

His explanations concerning the sources of possession, and how they infiltrate people, are of great interest to all involved in this work.

José Lacerda de Azevedo, M.D. was a medical doctor in Brazil who worked in a 'Spiritist Hospital' and developed a superior method of linking patients, discarnate doctors, and other helpers using mediums.

He explored the astral planes of existence to an unsurpassed degree, and wrote a book in Portuguese called 'Spirit and Matter' which detailed his experiences, with many case histories.

I have included extracts from his book covering the dark side of Heaven and how the souls of people who use black magic are subjected to extreme misuse and degradation in the astral, where their debts are 'called in' by the masters in charge of the dark forces.

Gwendolyn Awen Jones is a clairvoyant lady who was raped, had abortions, and then became a healer who concentrated on the effect that failure to be born (or early death in childhood) had not only on the parents (especially the mother) but also on the baby souls involved - an aspect not usually considered by exorcists or medical personnel.

Her book 'A Cry from the Womb' is full of case histories that demonstrate the detrimental effects on the mother in later life - from the failure to be born for whatever reason (or early childhood death) due to the influences from the deceased baby souls who still 'hang around' the mother and cause problems.

Gwendolyn's discourse on her perceptions of the human aura are extremely enlightening.

In discussion with Gwendolyn (and other mystics) it was considered probable that the intrusion of a discarnate baby soul into a conceived foetus already occupied by another baby soul could be an explanation for lesbian and gay people - where the intruding (and more powerful discarnate baby soul having a lifeline of one sex) takes command of the foetus of the opposite sex, over ruling the correct baby soul which has a lifeline of the opposite sex.

One of my own cases, when I was doing my best to help a pair of ladies who were lesbians, led to the discovery that the dominant lesbian lady had been one of a pair of twins; the other twin, a most powerful male baby soul, had died in the womb, and taken over his sister's mind and body.

He was so powerful that her body had been subjected to severe illnesses of all her female organs, most of which had then been removed surgically. He gained control of all her lesbian partners, causing havoc to them whenever they considered ending their part in the relationships that had developed.

It has been estimated that about 10% of the population are to some extent lesbian or gay - the intrusion of discarnate baby souls would account for this, especially since the religious ceremonials do not adequately handle the deaths in early childhood, and are completely non-existent if death occurs before birth.

In most cases I would not recommend that an exorcist removes such a dominant soul if the person has grown accustomed to the situation; but in the above case action had to be taken to lessen the power used by the intruder to hurt others.

Ho'oponopono is a Huna term which is fully described in that chapter, which tells of its use to heal inmates in an asylum - some who were vicious criminals.

The work was done at a distance, based on the files of those concerned, without the Healer ever meeting the inmates, and it was completely successful - a wonderful example of working in the Matrix.

Concerning Religions

Many exorcists seem to be associated with a religion. It is my experience that the darkest forces are not concerned with religions, which are probably rather poor human endeavours to understand the Spiritual worlds. My work is with the Angelic Beings (including enlightened souls) who are above, and has been very successful.

It is recognized by many religions, including the early Christians, that we have many lives, and that the effect of past lives does have an influence on our present life. These lives may well vary between different regions of this (and other) earths and so experience different religions.

The approach of many exorcists is to take out the possessing entities and send them away.

Unfortunately this allows them to re-infest others in the future. It is necessary to give these entities good healing and ensure that they are taken to their correct places - the healing to include removal of all their problems that cause them to infect others.

Holistic Exorcism is Teamwork

In all the works described by the sources that are mentioned in our research on successful exorcism it is the Angelic Beings and Souls in Heaven who do the work - the exorcist operates purely as a conduit or co-ordinator, requesting feedback from the entities via the person being healed.

I have found that my Heart is my link to these wonderful Beings - and can link to the Heart of the person being healed, working with their sub-conscious to identify and locate the causes of problems.

This link can be extended to the entities involved, usually via the sub-conscious, so that physical feedback from the person is no longer needed in doing the exorcism - but is most important in confirming that beneficial changes have occurred.

When a person requests assistance, all associated with them are checked for possession by dark forces so that more controllers are identified, located, and their slaves freed and healed. This has happened a number of times to those incarcerated in mental institutions, giving relief to others in these places.

It seems that most clairvoyants are unable to see the dark cord that connect the souls controlled by the dark forces to their controllers - and that this is so even with the Angelic Beings.

To overcome this, I understand that teams of the Soul Spirits of non-human life forms now work with the Angelic Beings and use their smelling and intuitive skills to identify these cords and trace them to the 'dungeons' and 'fortresses' ruled by the upper levels of the dark forces.

Teams of Spiritual Warriors then attack and demolish these places, removing the powers of the dark controllers, releasing captives, and sending all to be healed in the way that is best for all creation.

I consider it most dangerous to do any exorcism myself; any close encounter gives the possessing entities a chance to attack the exorcist. I am just a conduit for the help to be given, which is the work of the Angelic Beings, and I leave all contact to them.

I do this by asking my Heart to connect with the Angelic Beings and to give them guidance as needed, based on the parameters outlined in this book.

First watching teams are sent to the person to locate and identify the problems and their causes. When these are reported, I run through a check list to determine the identities, characteristics, and values of the entities involved. Then action is taken to make corrections and give healing.

This check list is completed using a Pendulum and indicator diagrams, and the progress of the work is watched using a Pendulum over my non-Dowsing hand - as I describe in detail in this book.

The check list is then repeated to record the changes as reported - feedback from the person is most valuable as a guide to one's accuracy and effectiveness, and in case of any additional possession taking place.

At the end I give energy to assist in the exorcism and healing by 4 deep 'HA' breathes, a method borrowed from Huna, and I send my love, gratitude and thanks to all who assisted in the exorcism.

Remember that having fear of entities results in giving them power. It is most important to be neutral - without any hate, anger, or fear. Consider that they have been hurt, and that the healing given is for these entities as well as for the person being attacked.

In October 2012 I was selected to be one of the Dowsers who spoke at the Dowsers World Summit; you can listen to my talk by downloading the recording:

www.dowsers.ca/WorldSummit.mp3

Namaste

I see in you myself
I recognize in you my image
We are all the same

I will help you in all you do with good intent
Without hurt or harm to others

Not for reward
But because it is the best way to be

To operate in True Holy Love, Namaste

Chapter 2

Advanced Clinical Experiences

Extracted from Dr. William Baldwin's article from Vol.4.1: Jan.-March 1995 of the Lifestream Letter

The Basis

Extensive contemporary clinical evidence suggests that discarnate beings, the spirits of deceased humans, can influence living people by forming a physical or mental connection or attachment, and subsequently imposing detrimental physical and/or emotional conditions and symptoms.

This condition has been called the 'possession state', 'possession disorder', 'spirit possession syndrome', 'spirit obsession', or 'spirit attachment'.

Earthbound spirits (usually the surviving consciousness of deceased humans) are the most prevalent possessing, obsessing or attaching entities to be found.

The disembodied consciousness seems to attach itself and merge fully or partially with the subconscious mind of a living person, exerting some degree of influence on thought processes, emotions, behavior and the physical body.

The entity becomes a parasite in the mind of the host. A victim of this condition can be totally amnesic about episodes of complete takeover.

A spirit can be bound to the earth plane by the emotions and feelings connected with a sudden traumatic death. Anger, fear, jealousy, resentment, guilt, remorse, even strong ties of love can interfere with the normal transition.

Erroneous religious beliefs about the afterlife can prevent a spirit from moving into the Light because the after death experience does not coincide with false expectations or preconceived notions of the way it is supposed to be.

Following death by drug overdose, a newly deceased spirit maintains a strong appetite for the drug, and this hunger cannot be satisfied in the non-physical realm. The being must experience the drug through the sensorium of a living person who uses the substance. This can only be accomplished through a parasitic attachment to the person. Many drug users are controlled by the attached spirit of a deceased drug addict.

Earth Bound Spirit

Many spirits remain in the earth plane due to a lack of awareness of their passing. At the time of death several choices are available for the newly deceased spirit. It can follow the direct path to the Light described in the near death experience (Moody, 1975; Ring, 1980); if there is an attached spirit the process may be more difficult. The newly deceased being can carry the attached earthbound to the Light thereby rescuing this lost soul. Often, the deceased is able to break away from the attached earthbound spirit and go to the Light alone.

After this separation occurs the earthbound can be lost again, wandering in the lower astral plane, often described as the gray place or the intermediate place. It can await the next incarnation of the being to whom it was attached. The entity can locate the being in the new incarnation and reconnect. This repeated attachment can occur for many lifetimes of the host. However, the earthbound can just as quickly attach to another unsuspecting person after separating from the former host at the time of death.

If the newly deceased spirit cannot break away from the attached spirit or hasn't strength enough to carry it into the Light, it can become earthbound also, with the original earthbound still attached to it. This pair can then attach to another living person. After death, the spirit of this person also may be prevented from reaching the Light due to the nested, or layered, attached spirits.

This spirit becomes part of the chain of earthbound spirits that can compound until it numbers in the dozens, even hundreds.

An attachment can be benevolent in nature, totally self serving, malevolent in intention, or completely neutral. Attachment to any person may be completely random, even accidental. It can occur simply because of physical proximity to the dying person at the time of the death. In about half the cases encountered in clinical practice it is a random choice with no prior connection in this or any other incarnation. In the remainder some connection can be found, some unfinished business from this or another lifetime.

Even if there is some prior interaction between the host and the attaching entity, the attachment only perpetuates the conflict and carries little possibility for resolution, though every experience has the potential for learning of some kind.

Most people are vulnerable to spirit attachment on many occasions in the normal course of life. Some investigators in this field estimate that between 70% and 100% of the population are affected or influenced by one or more discarnate spirit entities at some time in their life (Berg, 1984, p. 50; Fiore, 1987b).

Attracting Possession

Any mental or physical symptom or condition, strong emotion, repressed negative feeling, conscious or unconscious need can act like a magnet to attract a discarnate entity with the same or similar emotion, condition, need or feeling. Anger and rage, fear and terror, sadness and grief, guilt, remorse or feelings of the need for punishment can invite entities with similar feelings.

Severe stress may cause susceptibility to the influence of an intrusive spirit. Altering the consciousness with alcohol or drugs, especially the hallucinogens, loosens one's external ego boundaries and opens the subconscious mind to infestation by discarnate beings. The same holds true for the use of strong analgesics and the anesthetic drugs necessary in surgery.

A codeine tablet taken for the relief of the pain of a dental extraction can sufficiently alter the consciousness to allow entry to a spirit.

Physical intrusions such as surgery or blood transfusion can lead to an entity attachment. In the case of an organ transplant the spirit of the organ donor can literally follow the transplanted organ into the new body. Physical trauma from auto collision, accidental falls, beatings or any blow to the head can render a person vulnerable to an intrusive spirit.

The openness and surrender during sexual intercourse can allow the exchange of attached entities between two people. Sexual abuse such as rape, incest or molestation of any sort creates a vulnerability to spirit invasion. Violence during the sexual abuse increases the likelihood of intrusion by an opportunistic spirit.

Attachment

A living person can have dozens, even hundreds of attached spirits as they occupy no physical space. They can attach to the aura or float within the aura, outside the body. If any part of the body of the host has a physical weakness the earthbound can attach to that area because of a corresponding weakness or injury to the physical body of the spirit prior to death. A spirit can lodge in any of the chakras of the host, drawn by the particular energy of the chakra or by the physical structures of that level of the body.

Connection with an earthbound spirit may be established by the purposeful choice of either the spirit or the living human due to a strong emotional bond between them in this life or in a previous lifetime together.

A grieving person can welcome the spirit of a dear departed one only to find the consequences unbearable.

Effect of Attachment

A living human can be affected by an attached spirit in many different ways. The discarnate entity retains the psychic energy pattern of its own ailments following death and can produce in the host any mental aberration or emotional disturbance and any symptom of physical illness.

Erratic or inconsistent behavior can result from a shifting of control between separate entities. This behavior is similar in appearance to the phenomenon of switching between alters in multiple personality disorder (MPD).

This condition can be extremely confusing and frightening for a person and for their family.

An attached entity can be associated with any emotional track of a living person such as anger, fear, sadness or guilt. The emotional energy of the entity intensifies the expression of a specific emotion, often leading to inappropriate overreactions to ordinary life situations.

A subpersonality, that is a splinter or subordinate personality, can maintain a connection with an entity who came in at the chronological age when the subpersonality splintered away from the main personality due to a traumatic experience. The discarnate spirit may have joined at the time of the emotional trauma to help the child in the time of need. The continued connection with the entity prevents healing and integration of this subpersonality into the main personality system.

The mental, emotional and physical influence of an attached entity can alter the original path of karmic options and opportunities of the host.

It can disrupt the planned life line by hastening death or prolonging life, thus interfering with any specific checkout point.

An entity of the opposite gender can influence the sexual preference and gender brientation. An attached entity can influence the choice of marriage partners and the choice of a partner for an extra-marital affair.

Many areas of a person's life can be influenced by one or more attached entities. In short, spirit attachment can interfere with any aspect of the life of the unsuspecting host.

The host is usually unaware of the presence of attached spirits. The thoughts, desires and behaviors of an attached entity are experienced as the person's own thoughts, desires and behaviors. The thoughts, feelings, habits and desires do not seem foreign if they have been present for a long time, even from childhood. This is a major factor in the widespread denial of the concept and lack of acceptance of the phenomena of discarnate interference and spirit attachment, obsession or possession. This is equally true for people in general and for professional therapists.

Awareness of Attachment

In most cases, a person can only experience and acknowledge the reality of the condition after an attached entity has been released. The realization may come some months after a releasement session as the person suddenly notices the absence of a familiar attitude, desire, addiction or behavior.

The symptoms of spirit attachment can be very subtle. An attached spirit may be present without producing any noticeable symptoms. Yet attached entities always exert some influence ranging from a minor energy drain to a major degree of control or interference.

Complete possession and takeover can result in suppression of the original personality.

The earthbound spirit does not replace the rightful spirit in the body in such a case, it just usurps control.

An attached earthbound spirit cannot maintain life in a human body after the original spirit being has separated from the body in the transition of death.

A newly formed spirit attachment is usually more obvious to the unfortunate host. An attached entity can cause any of the following signs and symptoms: sudden onset of drug or alcohol usage; unusual and inappropriate speech, accent or foreign or unknown language, any behavior patterns inconsistent with normal conduct; unfamiliar reactions to familiar situations; repetitive and unusual movements of the body which are experienced as beyond one's control; unusual physical sensations or symptoms in the absence of a medically sound organic cause; loss of the normal sense of one's personal identity; a feeling that a spirit of some kind or another person has taken over control of one's mind and/or body; noticeable personality changes, however slight, following surgery, organ transplant, accident, emotional upset or moving into a new home.

As a result of a newly formed spirit attachment or possession, physical appetites for food, sex, alcohol or drugs can increase drastically. Personal attitudes and beliefs can suddenly change as can taste in clothing. The voice and even facial features and appearance can alter dramatically.

These sudden changes in behavior can be a factor in convincing the most skeptical person that there is an attached entity. Many people have the mistaken notion that there must be some bizarre outward signs caused by an interfering spirit such as depicted in the movie *The Exorcist,* based on the book of the same name (Blatty, 1971).

The movie depicted a true case, but some symptoms and behaviors of the girl actually came from two other cases, added for dramatic impact. Incidences of such violent possession are rare.

Is Permission Needed?

Spirit attachment does not require the permission of the host. This seems to be a violation of free will. It also appears to refute the popular notion that each person is totally responsible for creating his or her reality and that there are no victims.

The apparent conflict here stems from the definitions of permission and free will choice. Ignorance and denial of the possibility of spirit interference is no defense against spirit attachment. Belief or lack of belief regarding the existence of intrusive entities has no bearing on the reality of these beings and their behavior.

In denial and ignorance, most people do not refuse permission to these non-physical intruders.

Individual sovereign beings have the right to deny any violation or intrusion by another being. With limited, if any, knowledge and distorted perceptions of the nature of the spirit world, the non-physical reality, many people leave themselves open and create their own vulnerability as part of creating their own reality.

 It is fashionable today among many 'New Age' enthusiasts to attempt to channel some higher power, a spirit teacher or master who will use the voice mechanism of any willing person to speak 'words of wisdom'. Some use the terminology 'for my highest good' when calling for a spirit to channel through.

This activity constitutes permission and welcome for a discarnate spirit. The identifiers such as 'master' and 'teacher' and qualifiers such as 'for my highest good', will be claimed by the entities to be personally valid identifications, qualities or attributes.

Unfortunately, some opportunistic spirits who respond to this invitation refuse to leave at the end of the channeling session.

Dr Baldwin's Books

Dr Baldwin gives some detailed examples and case histories of his clinical experiences in his book 'Healing Lost Souls - Releasing Unwanted Spirits from your Energy Body' published by Hampton Roads, ISBN 987-1-57174-366-4.

Note that his work is primarily 'face to face' - or sometimes with his wife as a medium. He does not give any examples of distant exorcism.

His masterpiece is his book 'Spirit Releasement Therapy - A Technique Manual' published by Headline Books, ISBN 978-0-929915-16-6.   This   book   includes   a   deep appreciation of almost all that is involved in exorcism with detailed accounts of case histories. A 'Must Read' for all who do exorcism work !

Notes

Chapter 3

Spirit & Matter
- New Horizons For Medicine

Abstracted from the book by

José Lacerda de Azevedo, M.D.

Brilliant Brazilian Physician

THE ROOTS OF UNCERTAINTY.

For centuries, science was subordinate to the dogmas of the medieval scholastic. The moment it was freed from its static and anti-experimental chains - through arduous effort - during the Renaissance, and science began to employ objective research in the pursuit of liberty, and was victorious.

This victorious posture is still maintained today, but it is being wormeaten by biases that are as sticky as the dogmas that science faced in the old times.

It repels, with the disdain it showed the old inquisition and the same false superiority, all those who inform us about the unknown universe that exists beyond our three-dimensional universe.

The psychic sciences, for instance, while they are concerned with the mind, restrict their objectives exclusively to *living beings*; any other ontological *reality* has been discarded by scientists - who consider these experiments unreal and unlikely because they do not see nor feel them. All those phenomena that these ontological realities provoke in human beings, are studied on living brains and they are always linked to mental activities.

THE SEVEN BODIES

According to the septenary conception, the Spirit-Man is composed of two distinct strata: the Divine Triad, constituted by the "Christic I," and the "Inferior Quaternary," linked to the personality and which is mutable like it.

In these strata, each series or body has a denomination and distinct characteristics, specific functions and manifestations limited to the field or dimension to which it is linked, since each of these bodies vibrates in a distinct dimensional universe.

The Physical Body

The physical (somatic) body is the fleshy outer cover (envelope) in which we live - something similar to a diving suit: heavy and almost cumbersome, which we use in the physical environment.

It is composed of chemical compounds that are cleverly manipulated by the phenomenon called life.

In fact, there is life in each of these chemical elements. Everything inside us is life. We exist with our major life seated in a compound of a myriad of smaller lives that organize this compound.

As our body is made of Matter, it operates with ease in the physical environment since the body and the environment belong to the same electromagnetic dimension.

The Etheric Body

This body is of an extremely tenuous structure. It is invisible because it is diaphanous, of dense electromagnetic nature, but its wave length is superior to that of ultra-violet light. This is why the etheric body is easily disassociated by ultra-violet light when it is exuded by the physical body. It is quintessential, almost reaching immortality.

The physiological equilibrium reflects the harmony that prevails in the cosmos - the function of the etheric body is to establish health automatically, without interference of consciousness.

While it distributes vitalizing vitamins to the physical body, this equilibrium makes sure that the vital functions stay in balance and that the corporeal set maintains its harmonic equilibrium. In this way the physiological equilibrium promotes the healing of wounds, the cure of localized diseases, etc.

Functioning as a 'plastic' mediator between the astral body (the rougher body of the spirit) and the physical body, the body *or etheric double* is of material nature: it belongs to the domain of the flesh-man.

While the somatic body is composed of solids, liquids and gases that form cells, tissues and systems, the etheric body is constituted by the same elements and minerals; however, it is structured in such a tenuous state that it escapes totally from laboratory tests, unless the body is exteriorized and sufficiently condensed that it becomes visible and palpable in these abnormal conditions.

Although it seems to be a ghost, the etheric body is not spiritual and dissolves a few hours after death. Sometimes it can be seen at cemeteries, in the form of a light cloud that dissolves little by little. The etheric body does not have consciousness.

It can be vital food for the lower human spirits and for the immense variety of beings living in the astral - chiefly the zoologically inferior ones and those that visit cemeteries. Clairvoyants without experience quite often mix up the deactivated etheric doubles (crusts) with ghosts of the dead.

A great number of diseases that are considered settled in the human body, in reality have their seat in the anatomic substratum of the etheric organization. It is from there that they pass to the somatic body, where they appear as vital dysfunctions.

It is through the etheric structure that the volatile acts, desires, emotions, and any manifestation of the superior consciousness act upon the physical body, or more precisely on the physical brain.

The Astral Body

The spiritual covering nearest to Matter is called the astral body; it can easily be seen by clairvoyants. All spirits that embody in mediums have this subtle corporeal structure. It is as necessary for the manifestation of the spirit in the dimension in which it is (astral), as the body is necessary for human beings.

It is within this body that the spirits live in the astral dimension; in those that usually communicate in spiritual sessions, this vehicle is rather dense (the density is according to the evolutionary degree of the possessor). Those that do not have it anymore, because they are more developed, communicate with the mediums by mental syntony (a synchronous joining) without embodiment.

The spirits that are very materialized live in erraticity, together with the incarnated beings.

Erraticity is the existential state without any useful or objective goal, a state in which some disincarnated spirits exist.

Although the primordial cause of this state is the ignorance of its own evolution and the spirit's role in the cosmic context, this anguishing existential perplexity gets worse with the occurrence of other factors.

These include: ignorance and hopelessness about the possibility of evolution; addiction to material goods, to people, etc.; continuous revolt for considering oneself impotent to rule over nature, as the incarnated do; the natural difficulties of adapting to the environment, the distortions of evaluation, and the many personal, moral and material factors that disturb the recently disincarnated.

If these erratic spirits are not too perverse, they can easily be taken to recovery stations that exist in the astral. To do this, it is only necessary to orient them firmly.

Together with orientation, we can use a faster way to convince them. If we first treat and clean them, change their clothes, heal and cure their diseases, wounds and pains, even the most ignorant and inflexible ones will become hopeful and decide to develop by working and learning.

This change in attitude is very understandable. Spirits without any evolution are used to remaining in the states of suffering that made them die, and so they go on living, sometimes in intense pain for many years.

When they get rid of this awful prolonging of their agony (and this can happen in only a few minutes through the use of strong jets of healing Energy as we soon will see) these poor creatures open up to love.

While the spirits develop, they lose their astral body little by little, becoming more and more diaphanous as seen by clairvoyants. After some time, undergoing evolution, they lose the astral body completely, keeping only the subtler spiritual coverings. But all the perispiritual coverings are also abandoned at a certain time, until only the Pure Spirit is left in.

Under certain circumstances, artificial or natural, the astral body can separate from the physical body, by taking with it all the other coverings and even its own spirit. This normally happens while the person is asleep, when he loses consciousness and the vital functions are lowered to a minimum level necessary for metabolic exchanges.

Many sensitives can easily get out of their bodies, in spontaneous trances. But this can also happen to other people, in pathological or special occasions, as for instance, a strong emotional shock, debility due to long periods of sickness, voluminous hemorrhaging, surgical shocks and other traumatic conditions.

People can go to distant places, they can describe these places, evaluate their actions and those of others, they can have physical sensations, everything in perfectly conscious conditions - thanks to the connection with the physical brain, through the silver string.

The spirit remains attached to the body, independently of its distance from the body, by means of the silver string. If it gets torn up, however, death occurs. It is irreversible.

One of the most important functions of the astral body is sensitivity. We know that it resides in this field or body; the physical body only transmits received stimuli; the record of painful or pleasant sensations is up to the structure.

Vices are of a psychic nature exactly due to this fact; their origin is in the astral: it is the astral that feels. For this reason we take our vices and passions with us when we die; if it were otherwise, there would be no reason for the disincarnated to go on suffering physical pains, or carry painful deformations with them - as has been verified in spiritual sessions.

Sensation is the roughest form of feelings. It is primary, instinctive. Emotion is much more complex, it is linked to desire; it can be exacerbated until it reaches the abnormality of passion. We cannot forget that sensations, like emotions, are very important states of our consciousness, since they give color and power to our acts.

Our astral body constantly loses energy, needing, therefore, an energy supply for its sustenance, similar to feeding the physical body. But the nature of this food varies very greatly; it goes from protein broth for the more materialized spirits, provided by the astral assistance stations, to quintessential energies that feed the superior spirits, which are gathered (through prayers) directly from the infinite reservoir of cosmic energy.

The Mental Body

The mental body is the vehicle that uses the cosmic 'I' to manifest itself as a concrete and abstract intellect; it is in this body that the will gets transformed into action, subsequent to choosing the volitional act.

It is a field of elaborated reasoning, from which the powers of mind, the phenomena of cognition, memory, and the evaluation of our acts, surge because it is the seat of the manifested active consciousness.

While physical sensibility and emotions flow from the astral body, the mental vehicle can be considered the source of the intellect.

In a certain way, the mental body is still an inferior covering, because it is a consequence of these phenomena or functions that conventionally are called 'intellect'. Only on superior levels of consciousness, where the virtues that result from affective love for all beings are present at their highest degree, can the highest spirituality, which is our essence, manifest itself.

This field, body or dimension of the Spirit-Man can be divided in two, for a better understanding:

1. Concrete mental body, also called the inferior mental body: it deals with simple, quite objective perceptions, e.g., the ones of material objects, people, houses, vehicles, etc.

2. Abstract mental body, causal body or superior mental body: it elaborates and structures principles and abstract ideas ad infinitum; it is the process responsible for scientific and technological advances, and also for our entire philosophic foundation.

The mental body has an approximately ovoid form that involves the physical body. Its peripheral portions constitute the aura, and the aura is of varied color and size according to the frequency of the vibratory fields generated by thoughts.

It is easy for clairvoyants to perceive what is going on in the minds of people: good thoughts are of light, crystalline, brilliant colors; the inferior ones (hatred, envy, vengeance, etc.), are of dark, dense and unpleasant colors. The aura, consequently, reveals the tonic note of the mental field of a person.

The mental Energy can be projected into Space, by means of structures known as thought forms.

They consist of an energy nucleus that has its form modeled by the mind that projects it; they can harm or benefit a person, according to the will of the person who creates it - consciously or unconsciously.

The negative ones take the form of darts, arrows, projectiles, or turbid fields, for example.

The positive ones, more efficient, take the form that the operator wants them to have; we can, for instance, use the mental energy also to benefit disincarnated spirits, by cleaning and dressing them and giving them food, with the objective of improving their spiritual conditions.

The natural field of this energy is the mental field. When projected, this energy normally acts first on the mental field or body of other beings, and from there it goes (already converted to psychomotor actions) to the astral and etheric bodies or fields.

The Buddhic Body

There is almost nothing to be said about the vibratory structure (or field, body or dimension), closest to the spirit. This body is so distant from our physical standards, and from our means of expression, that it is not possible to compare it by describing it.

It is possible to say that buddhi is the perispirit according to the etymological acceptance of the word: it is the first vibratory structure that, by involving the spirit, demonstrates it in an active way.

However, a short time ago, we were allowed to discover an interesting property of this structure that can be used, and in a very practical way, in the treatment of the incarnated and disincarnated - since both are, first of all, spirits.

As this body is timeless (as the superior mental body is, too), we used the technique to reach this superior dimension of people, as a starting point to scrutinize their pasts. In this way we could detect anomalous situations, very painful events, deeply rooted in time, in the extremely tenuous stratum of a hidden past that happened at very remote times.

The Atmic Body

Also called the 'Essence Spirit'. Through millennia and successive civilizations, any attempt to describe what we designate by 'spirit' is considered incomplete because of the inefficacy of words.

The concepts of Vedic Philosophy continue to be enlightening due to their transparency. According to the Vedas, the One and Universal Being - Brahma (The Non-manifested), transcendent and eternal - becomes immanent in his temporary action, when he manifests himself.

The beings that he emanates, contain his essence, in the same way as the thinker is in his thoughts. The absolute, the universal, is manifested in each individualized being, even in the very small ones, exactly because it is absolute, and, therefore, escapes human understanding, it transcends whatever exists.

This omnipresent absolute, manifested and manifesting in each being, is called Atman or Spirit. The pure atmic 'body' or 'Spirit', this 'Cosmic I', constitutes the Divine Essence in each created being. We are all identical to God in the sense of Being (Essence), but different from Him.

The Chakras

The chakras are power centers, real vortices through which the dynamic magnetic fields are linked to the physical body. The seat of the chakras is in the etheric double, but their origin is in superior structures; these energies in vortices are of a cosmic nature and spiritually feed the being that manifests the phenomenon life.

Always rotating, they have varying angular velocity, depending on their location in superior or inferior areas of the body.

Chakras are organs which belong to the transcendental physiology of the human being.

They are fulcrums of power actively animated, and continuously receive fluxes of cosmic and other energies from outside the body. These energies are transformed by the chakras, lowering the frequency, according to the type of chakra. After the energies have been duly modulated, they are distributed in the areas or fields where the chakras act.

APOMETRIA.

The term Apometria is composed of the Greek word apo, which means 'beyond' and metron, 'measurement'. The unfolding is essentially the separation of the astral (or mental) body from the physical body.

In 1965 a man showed up at the Spiritist Hospital of Porto Alegre, saying that he had a technique for medical treatment, totally different from official medicine: he used the service of disincarnated doctors who indicated the therapeutics for the illnesses of sick people. The man was called Luiz Rodrigues, from Puerto Rico; he had been living for many years in Rio de Janeiro.

At first sight, his technique did not seem to be any different from the mediumistic processes of Kardecian Spiritism, although he insisted he was not a follower of this Doctrine. But it proved to be very different!

Instead of the disincarnated doctors coming to the patient, it was the patient who, unfolded, went to the doctors of the astral, to get his diagnosis and therapeutics.

Mr. Rodrigues simply used a slow, regressive counting, starting with the number corresponding to the age of the patient. When the counting was done, the patient was out of his body.

The technique of apometria unfolding proved to be applicable to any kind of person independent of age, health, mental state, or even the resistance that the person could offer.

Once the acting energy comes from outside, it does not depend on the person's will. Easy to use, Apometria is of unquestionable efficiency.

The greatest success of Apometria is in its application to mediums who achieve easier contact with the spiritual world.

In our work we use clairvoyant mediums who when they are unfolded can see in the astral field. Other people, without clairvoyance, do not even believe that they are unfolded. On the other hand, experienced mediums can see and hear spirits during the trances of unfolding. In addition, they can move in space where they visit astral colonies, perform efficient work to redeem suffering spirits, and participate in organized aid caravans in that dimension; they also visit incarnated sick people in their homes, integrating spiritual groups whose objective is the cleansing of homes.

To assist a sick person we use unfolded mediums in contact with the doctors of the astral. Next, we unfold the sick person, too, who is then, in his astral body, assisted by the disincarnated doctors in the presence of the unfolded mediums.

These, then, relate everything that is going on while the doctors take care of the sick - diagnostics, astral surgeries, details of the patients problems - with the elucidation of the disease and practical orientations for the consolidation of the cure. Unfolded, the patients are assisted with more efficiency, depth, and speed by the disincarnated doctors.

The diagnostics used are very detailed and precise; in astral surgeries, it is common to use high techniques and sophisticated equipment in hospitals of the superior astral.

This description - dead doctors treating the sick astral body, mediums and patients visiting invisible hospitals, with surgery rooms and advanced equipment (and, of course, buildings, gardens, vehicles, etc.) - all seems to be fanciful imagination, as if it were scientific fiction. But it is not.

For more that twenty years, dozens of mediums have unfolded at the Love and Charity Hospital, the astral institution that helps us in our spiritual work. During all this time different mediums (first separately, and then in groups) and on different days, contributed much to our careful investigation, giving identical descriptions of the gardens where they rested, of the building, the rooms, the surgical centers, allowing us an accurate examination of the surgical techniques.

The Obsessors

Dr Lucerda uses this term to mean those who are obsessed with causing hurt to others. The use of 'magnetized' may indicate a very close attachment.

Almost without exception, patients come followed by a group of obsessors: the spiritual agents of their diseases. We have to assist, first, these unhappy spirits, some of whom are in great suffering and have been magnetized to the sick for a long time. They do not limit themselves to persecuting their victims all the time: they try to harm them in all possible forms; their vengeance is blind. Usually they are enemies who had been victims of their present victims in former incarnations.

The obsessors act individually, in small groups, or in large gangs - it depends on the magnetization they have with the victim, their degree of peril, the astral means they have, their intelligence and mental potentiality. In any event, they are terrifying.

Once they are gathered, they have to be taken to specialized hospitals in the astral or to the regions the Guiding Spirits send them according to the vibratory standard of each sufferer. Giving them love offers them an understanding of hatred and its dark consequences.

We learned that we can never leave an obsessor free. They seldom have their behavior and attitudes modified in Spiritist sessions which use only dialectics to enlighten them.

Usually more than one session is needed to convince them. They cannot easily change the cruel behavior they are used to, particularly if they are evildoers working for incarnated or disincarnated entities who are interested in the destruction of a person.

In the haste and desire to harm, obsessors use highly refined techniques of torture to harass their victims. They put all kinds of instruments on the victim's bodies (ropes, chains, lacerating fetters, etc - as thought forms) to weaken them and cause continuous suffering. Therefore, mysterious illnesses occur, with baffling symptoms, that mislead medical diagnoses.

Among the many new syndromes that Apometria allowed us to discover, we can cite the diseases caused by parasitic devices fixed in the nervous system of the astral body of the sick. This syndrome, for its importance, could stand beside the classic syndromes of medicine; however it is provoked by technicians of darkness, interested in harming people physically and mentally.

Apometria causes real miracles in the treatment. Not only do those being obsessed receive treatment, the obsessors also are given treatment, either individually or in small groups.

Importance of Mental Energy

The 'Open Sesame' for the world of the spirits, the magic key to actuate this dimension parallel to ours, is mental energy impelled by an act of will, by a firm and objective will that is transformed into power.

We must realize that it is the same volitional act that actuates and gives us power over the physical world, an act that is in the origin of the conquests of every civilization.

The action of mental energy is not significantly different in the incarnated or disincarnated spirit. The alteration seems to be only a factor of time. In the physical world, everything takes more time to be constructed, since it is necessary to overcome the matter and the inertia of the mass. In the astral world, everything is faster.

This acknowledgment and the constant practical exploration of these open possibilities, in dealing with the spirits, constitute the secrets of the success that we have had so far in assisting them.

When we assist obsessors we do not care only about them. As we have already mentioned (and now do again to emphasize the fact), we also take care of their accomplices, because they never act by themselves - they usually are in the company of spirits of the same level of evolution. If we helped only the obsessor, we believe that our work would be incomplete, since we would leave an indefinite number (sometimes a very large number) of suffering and needy entities without assistance.

Life after Death

Note that every man keeps, on the other side of life, the same consciousness that animated him when he was alive: the same vices, the same defects, egotism, impulses of aggression and violence. No one becomes a saint just because he died.

When freed from flesh, individuals go on behaving as spirits, according to the old standards they had when they were alive - if not worse - in a degradation that is much more common than we imagine.

If, before death, the person was feeding feelings of hatred and vengeance, the moment he is disincarnated he will attack his enemy with all the means and power he has.

Not all interference is malicious; sometimes the spirit sees the patient, feels the beneficent vital aura that attracts him, because it makes him feel well. However, if the spirit is sick, he transfers his anguish and suffering to the incarnated.

Often the spirit does not want, deliberately, to harm the target-person. It is the consequence of an egotistic action of a being that makes another one the object of his care, and wishes ardently to make this target-person his. He demands that the other person obey his orders, blindly wanting to protect her, guide her, and with this kind of coercion, he impedes her enjoyment of a normal and healthy life with her fellow beings.

Real Obsession

Real obsession always implies a conscious and volitional action, with a clear objective, aiming at well-defined results and effects; the obsessor wants and knows very well what he is doing.

This premeditated action, planned and executed with great carefulness and sophistication, constitutes the great cause of psychic diseases.

Most of the pernicious actions of spirits upon the incarnated involve an extensive process that has been developing through Time and Space, where the pernicious and hateful action (the cause of the disease) is nothing but the continuous flux of charging mutual debts, perpetuating the suffering of both.

The persecutors of yesterday are the victims of today, in an interminable settlement of accounts, gloomier than dramatic.

Many obsessors act with the means they have, without any major knowledge of the spiritual world's laws. They try to destroy the enemy with clubs, whips, ropes, and similar tools, they wrap him with cables, fetters, ties, sweat cloth, etc.

The technique of fencing in the victim by various kinds of obsessions is another characteristic of complex obsession. The sick finds himself hemmed in, undefended, at the mercy of the disincarnated enemies and predators.

Through a well-detailed planning, (a plan of a really devilish plot, of the general staff, executed with military rigor) the technicians of evil investigate the victim's whole life, discover and 'convoke' all his disincarnated enemies to take revenge and destroy their foe.

The worst type of obsession is without doubt everything that involves the ominous black magic. When we face this kind of case, we know beforehand: a very critical treatment is going to be necessary to eliminate the (many) obsessors.

Overcoming Obsession

The first step is to deactivate the 'magnetic' fields, without this procedure, they would be going on acting indefinitely upon the victim.

This is very important because the 'magnetic' action only disappears if deactivated by an external action in relation to the person, or if the sick is able to increase his vibratory standard in such a way that it allows him to get rid of the 'magnetic' prison, by himself.

The actions of the sorcerers of Darkness are very well-known: deceitful, dissimulating, devilish - intelligent and experienced professionals of evil.

They received huge powers when they were initiated in temples of the past: they swore solemnly to use them only for good, but, in the course of time, due to immaturity and complex circumstances, they fell into decay.

The pure, wise men became practitioners of evil, caught in the trap of sexual passions, thirst for mean vengeance, or cupidity for richness and power.

Their acquired knowledge and powers are, therefore, at the service of sinister purposes. Their appalling actions embrace the world of human beings, and of the astral, too, where they have enormous, well-equipped bases.

To dominate a sorcerer, it is necessary to deprive him of his powers. But these can only be annulled by reconnecting him to the past, projecting him in a different equation of time.

Once he is deprived of his powers gained in initiation, the next step is the reduction of his mental potency.

If this is not done well, the chances to dominate him will be quite reduced. To succeed in their reduction, several techniques of corroborated efficacy have been used, which are applied according to the power and knowledge of the sorcerer.

After this - and only afterwards - we reach the most important step: we open the route of reincarnation for these spirits; reincarnation they have avoided by using their potent mental magnetism. We met some that had not reincarnated since their last existence in ancient Egypt - or even before.

Although these spirits may pretend to be very gentle, we should not be deceived by appearances which, in fact, hide their certainty that they are powerful and very clever in the practice of evil.

Dungeons of Darkness

In the spiritual world, mainly in the inferior zones of the Umbral (the lowest part of the astral plane), there proliferate large organized colonies of powerful sorcerers of Darkness. They imprison a great number of disincarnated spirits, enslaving them in a typical obsession. When we destroy colonies and bases directed by Darkness, it is necessary, first, to save the slaves.

Special attention has to be given to the electronic devices and/or parasites in the nervous system of the victim. This obsessive process implies specialized knowledge and sometimes complex, sophisticated techniques.

Reverse Obsession

Apparently very strange is the obsession of a mortal upon a disincarnated spirit. It seems paradoxical that a man can act upon a spirit. Nevertheless, this happens more frequently than we imagine, showing that the universes of the living and of the dead are interlinked.

As the mind of an incarnated man vibrates always in the spiritual world, the environment in which the spirit constantly lives (incarnated or not), this exchange becomes easy.

Chiefly during sleep, the incarnated can detach from matter and live, temporarily, in the spiritual world. In this way, a great deal can happen between alive and dead spirits, with exchanges of physical and even sexual sensations.

Once, when we assisted a woman, we faced an extremely restless and despairing spirit.

Since we thought that it was a simple obsession, we tried to convince him to abandon the one that we considered his victim. To our surprise he supplicated:

Look, if you can free me from this woman I will be very thankful to you. I have already done everything. But I cannot get rid of her!

But, how come that you are so subjugated, my dear, if you are a spirit with an immense possibility to follow your way of peace?

It is because you do not know the power of this witch. In my previous life she made me get married to her. It was a disastrous marriage, economically as much as morally. When I died I thought I was free of her. But what a deception! One day I was violently attracted by her. And I could never again get rid of her. When she sleeps she always calls me. More than that, she pulls me with an irresistible force. Please, for heaven's sake, free me from her.

We did what the spirit asked us. We freed him and conducted him to the station of recuperation.

A deeper study of the sick revealed that she had been a sorceress in the remote past. She sold oracles and magic filters for sorcery. She also practiced black magic. Now she was suffering from psychic and spiritual disturbances, caused by several entities that were charging her past debts.

The spirit that she had dominated was her former mate; in her previous life she married him, under the effect of a black magic work that was still acting upon her.

Obsession is also quite common among living people. All of us know dominating, despotic and egotistic individuals, who command the whole family, obligating everybody to do what they want. This kind of obsession, interfering even in the effectiveness of others, is nothing other than a case of obsession that is disguised in protectionism.

The classic real obsession is where the disincarnated spirit disturbs the incarnated one in every sense, to take revenge. The treatment is usually very difficult. The contender's affective problems take us to aberrant states of consciousness, so deeply do they root in violence and hatred, and with a perseverance that can be measured in centuries.

<u>Notes</u>

Chapter 4

APOMETRIC EXPERIENCES

When we were assisting a sick person at the Spiritist Hospital of Porto Alegre, we faced a painful case of obsession. Victim and torturer were alternating mutual persecution.

Sometimes one, sometimes the other one, got incarnated. And the one who incarnated suffered the action of the enemy that was still in the astral. To find a clue, we had to go backwards in time, stage by stage, through six past incarnations. Everything started in the Middle Ages, when one of them had been a servant and had suffered serious offenses inflicted by the feudal owner.

Implanted Devices

For years we have been observing, in sick people assisted at the 'Garden House', the presence of small and strange devices placed with exactness and great skill in the astral counterpart of the nervous system.

To clairvoyants they look as if they were attached to the physical body, since the astral body is superimposed on it. As this spiritual body is of the same physiology as the physical one, any disturbance in its functioning will fatally affect it in a short time.

Ordinarily these devices are very tiny; and the people who are in a condition to see them seldom know about the anatomic details of the nervous system.

The objective of these electronic inventions (yes, electronic and sophisticated), is to cause functional disturbances in sensory, perceptual or motor areas, and in other nerve centers such as the nuclei of the cerebral base and of vegetative life.

The most common technique is to attach this device to the cerebrum or to the bones of the skull, using special screws. Afterwards they link the device by means of very thin filaments to different areas of the central nervous system or to the nuclei along the medulla, according to the desired objective.

We realized that some devices receive electromagnetic signals of controlled and variable intensity. Altering the entrance of physiological responses to normal stimuli, they emitted anomalous and sudden commands to the auditory area, for example; they suggested forms of self-destruction and compelled the subject to perform a variety of abominable and whimsical actions, injected directly into the cerebrum.

It is lamentable that in these cases physicians are almost unable to help. They cannot even console the patient because they do not believe what he says.

They classify the clinical state as an 'auditory hallucination' - a state that exactly, because it is an hallucination, does not exist for medicine!

Poisoned Objects

According to our experience, it is common to have obsessors put poisoned objects in open incisions during surgeries to cause the sick to feel the worst pain possible. By doing this, they impede cicatrization or cause, for example, the formation of dangerous, persistent fistulas in hollow viscera.

For this purpose they use wooden wedges, imbued with poisonous vegetal juices - everything is done in the astral world, but it reflects immediately on the physical body: pains, intense itching, disagreeable local heat, inflammation, etc. We have observed hundreds of cases with this type of pathology.

In our assistance we take out any harmful material and burn it with cosmic energy in the astral plane.

In the meanwhile, disincarnated doctors remove fistulas, do cleansing curettage, etc., and frequently treat the wounds with vegetal sap.

In 1985 we took care of a young lady - a newlywed - who presented a persistent cystitis along with genital dysfunction. Doctors attributed the functional disturbances to her recent wedding. But as the lady got worse, they decided to give her more profound tests and a specific treatment. The medicine was not very efficacious - it only lessened the symptoms.

Suffering from polaciuria (frequent urination, small quantity), dysuria (pain when urinating) and urinary incontinence, the patient felt very uncomfortable when she was with others.

When the apometric unfolding was done, we found a little object made of black wood that had been introduced deep into her uterus; and another one, similar to the first, was enlarging the vesical sphincter.

The process was to prevent pregnancy, to cause dysfunction due to the poison, and to provoke urinary incontinence.

We captured the obsessor. In a previous existence he wanted to win her love. He was despised by her and not well treated by her servants, because, although he was married, he went on trying to conquer her. Due to the bad treatment he received from the servants, he fractured a leg which did not heal well and so he became lame. He swore to take revenge but he only got it after death. He was able to close in on the woman he loved and who had incarnated again.

We discovered that the two had been partners in criminal activities in former incarnations. In the last one, the victim caused an abortion, the result of a clandestine love affair with the present obsessor. Consequently her genital field became vulnerable to spiritual evildoers, even to the less skillful ones.

Karmic Influences

There was a patient with a psychic process of chronic characteristics that made her feel rather sick, neurotic, full of fears, constantly worried with diseases. Although the patient was young, she showed early aging. She had already undergone innumerable spiritual treatments.

She was apometrically unfolded and had her vibratory frequency opened, but we did not detect any kind of obsessor. We decided, then, to investigate her karmic problem; so, we opened vibratory fields of the past.

We were surprised when we discovered that the patient had lived in ancient Egypt and, in an incarnation of that time, she suffered an intense action of black magic for various reasons.

In one of her lives she was very rich and had great political power, gaining powerful enemies who wanted to annihilate her. She still had them attached to her astral body.

We have already seen that obsession, usually, aims at making the obsessed suffer as much as possible until he dies. But among the cases we assisted there were many in which the obsessors did not want the victim's death, they wanted him to suffer as long as possible. In other cases, not so frequent, they want to harm him morally: they want their enemies to undergo the same sufferings that they inflicted upon the obsessors, in the past.

'Two Faced' Obsession

We have met obsessors that help their victims, in all possible ways to get very rich and to live in great comfort, playing an important role in society. In the last of these cases we assisted, the persecutor was enjoying himself very much with the moral suffering of his enemy. He was wealthy, he had a large group of friends, but was involved in all kinds of moral problems. His first-born son was an oligophrenic microcephalic. The oldest daughter followed the route of modern vices: she became drug addicted; she was also in favor of free love and even ended up stealing. Another son, maladjusted, became a homosexual, besides being addicted to drugs.

Even the man's wife, extremely voluptuous, was made to be disloyal to her husband. It is easy to imagine how bitter and full of disappointment the life of this man was, in spite of all his wealth and economic and social power.

Power Corrupts

Individuals who, in the past, for example, exerted positions of command, (kings, rulers, despotic military officers) incarnate with twisted mentality, demanding immediate assent to their opinions, if not total obedience. Vices that result from economic power are also very common and difficult to eradicate; our physical existence is energized and controlled by money.

There are also those important people and intellectuals, with messianic tendencies, who want to lead the crowd by means of forms of governments unacceptable for our historical moment; they usually are those politicians and demagogues that still are longing to be different from the common mortal, and who - according to them - have the right and the obligation to orient other people.

The number of these states of consciousness is so enormous that is it impossible to describe them in detail. We realized, however, that a good part of these stigmatized people (chiefly those who can have a certain influence upon others) is manipulated by the spirits of Darkness who, due to the lack of vigilance that characterizes them, tend to join in profound symbiosis of varied degrees.

We have met people who do not appreciate social life. They are misanthropes. After deeper investigation we find that they had been hermits or monks who spent their whole lives running from living with other people because of a fear of the sins of the flesh.

Usually these monks incarnate into the same sex, but they are always fleeing women. They are shy, naïve and unable to live in brotherly togetherness. They lived as recluses for many years, imprisoned and coerced in conceptions that marked their personality for a long time. With these antecedents, they easily become maladjusted. They do not know how to live in society.

At other times, we have met formerly powerful individuals who today feel frustrated in their impotence since they incarnated without splendor and power. They now are poor and tied to jobs that they hate; and besides this, they are persecuted by their disincarnated enemies.

According to all this, we can understand the terrible drama of humankind.

Almost all human beings are spiritually sick!

Mediumistic Problems

Years ago, we had a very interesting case.

One of our fellows, a good mediumistic potential and with several years of work in our group, was receiving a higher entity whose function was the one of a physician in the Love and Charity Hospital, in the astral. She syntonized perfectly with the spirit and received from him safe orientation for the sick's treatment and also for the unfolding techniques.

In the course of time, however, she started dominating the supervisor, making her personal opinions prevail about the best way to treat the sick.

At the beginning, we realized slight signs of animism in the disincarnated physician's communications - signs that suddenly appeared in the exaggerated emphasis of concepts that coincided with those of the medium. At this point the message was not yet distorted. There was only a strong stress on the aspects that were to the medium's interest, with an emotion that did not come from the communicating spirit.

The development of animism can be quite subtle as can be the trap in which a medium can be caught when not humble and vigilant. *Perhaps ego is a closer translation.*

Our fellow medium overlaid on the real message her own emotional opinion, reinforcing certain images and exaggerating some facets. But, as time went by, the undue interference got worse until there was a notorious mixture of her opinions with those of the spirit.

When the mediumistic-animistic jumble reached about 50% of animism, the unavoidable happened. The spirit, through the medium herself, (in an unquestionable authenticity) suspended the attention he gave to the sick because the assistance he was giving the medium was over.

Consequently, we lost a worker who could still be in service if she had cultivated humbleness. Unfortunately, it was not the only case at the Garden House.

Spiritual Parasiticism

As common as parasitism is among living beings, it is also extremely widespread among spirits. There are cases in which the spirit is not conscious of what he is doing; sometimes he even does not know that he has disincarnated. Other spirits, living only a vegetative life, parasitize a mortal without knowing what they are doing; they do not have the faintest idea about it; they are sick, disincarnated spirits in painful situations. Most of the cases are of unconscious parasitism.

But there are also parasites that are placed by obsessors; unconscious, sick spirits are linked to the incarnated's astral body, to weaken him. These situations happen frequently in cases of complex obsession, chiefly when the patient is abnormally debilitated.

The first step of the treatment is the separation of the parasite from the host. Then the care of the spirit follows; during his treatment, valuable elements can surge, making the incarnated individual's cure easier. Finally, we energize the host, and indicate conditions and prophylactic procedures to him.

Vampirism is the phenomenon in which a being, according to legends, leaves the tomb at night, to suck the blood of living people.

Vampirism, however, is not only practiced by beings that look like bats. There is a variety of vampires, from incarnated creatures to disincarnated parasites. All inferior spirits, idle and primary, can vampirize or parasitize dead and alive beings.

In both parasitism and vampirism, the suction of other being's energies occurs. But the difference is in the intensity of the ominous action, determined by the consciousness and cruelty with which it is practiced. The parasite usually causes less harm because he generally does not know what he is doing. Now, the real vampire is totally conscious of what he is doing and never spares a vampirized victim.

In 1985, we treated a case of advanced parasitism, in which the parasite was so tied to the victim that the clairvoyants did not perceive his presence. His astral body was so tightly bound to the incarnated creature's body that he could not be distinguished by common clairvoyants. He was only discovered when we unfolded the patient apometrically.

When he was unfolded, he carried the parasite with him - who, then, was immediately seen by the unfolded mediums.

We considered the case so interesting that we decided to investigate more deeply the spiritual problems. We induced the parasite to embody in a medium so we could question him.

It was an extremely long-suffering spirit, very hungry, since this was the state in which he disincarnated.

So great was his anguish and fear, he could not eat anything, he clung to us looking for shelter, and asked us to allow him to stay with us as he stayed with the sick person.

To make him feel relaxed we agreed. We even projected strong vital energy currents to feed him. He was very satisfied, but when we told him that he was going to leave the sick person, he clung more strongly to us, imploring us to allow him to suck our vital forces.

Some visitors who were present at our work became afraid. However, the spiritual parasite did not have any malefic intention. He felt very upset due to the lack of food, marked by a very painful incarnation. His primary vitiation obsessed him so; the only reason for his existence was the search for food.

For him, disincarnated as he was, any vital energy was valuable. and he was going to get it from any incarnated being that would shelter him.

Black Magic

Quite often we see sensitive people - mainly young people - suffering from low level obsessive processes (including black magic) that had not been directed specifically against them. They were affected only because they were near the true target.

These people become disturbed, anguished, stop working, feel sick and, in short, suffer the whole malefic action of the negative vibrations discharged against another person of their family, their home or their environment.

The true targets, however, are immune to that kind of spiritual attack or they are only slightly affected. The cause of this phenomenon is the great sensitivity of these extemporaneous receivers, who, without wanting to, enter in resonance with the negative torrents. In this way, they are used as a protective shield for the main target of these forces who usually is the head of the family.

In a process of black magic, we consider two situations:

<u>First:</u> The mobilization of natural forces chosen, manipulated and directed to harm the victim.

This is done by skillful artisans of Darkness, specialists in producing disharmony and suffering. Their objective is to destroy the victim, mentally or physically, through disorderly vibration of magnetic fields of extremely low frequency.

<u>Second:</u> The presence of one or more members of a group of low mental, intellectual, or spiritual level entities, some of who behave as slaves, constrained by other forces; others freely and conscientiously enjoy serving - with perverse ferocity - the 'Dragons of Evil'.

These low level entities are linked to the 'evil deeds' of the technicians of Darkness, incarnated or disincarnated. The slaves are used to watch the negative field and to whip the victim's astral body occasionally, besides leading those recently disincarnated (suffering and desperate) spirits close to the victim, transforming them into enormous vampires that the victim has to feed with his already meager energies.

Once the technicians and chiefs of the gang are captured, it is necessary to deactivate their bases in the Umbral - the lowest reaches of the astral plane.

Citadels of Darkness

The bases shelter many creatures and sometimes they are so big that they constitute a real citadel of Darkness. There are schools with regular classes to create technicians. It is there that they elaborate, well and safely, their plans to harass the incarnate.

Very well protected, these bases have abundant materials (often very sophisticated) to act directly or indirectly upon their victims - by means of all kinds of electronic devices, chiefly an arsenal of potent electromagnetic emitters, used to torment and annihilate human beings.

Their sources of energy are nuclear power plants situated deep under the constructions, placed there to avoid any outside invasion. These nuclear power plants provide energy for the various laboratories, specialized in all the imaginable and unimaginable branches of scientific experimentation.

We found, for instance, bases that specialized in the nervous system. They had models of brains of human beings and other primates, in large sizes, which were technically perfect and would be the envy of researchers on Earth.

Some time ago we found a base that was specialized in ... Cardiology! It was the only one we found, so far, with this kind of specialization. In one of the many meeting rooms there was an enormous heart on a table.

The heart was made of diaphanous material, where one could very clearly see the venous and arterial nets, and the whole nervous structure. The two mediums who had gone down to deactivate the base were surprised at the perfection of the model.

Specialists, the technicians of this umbraline model, used their knowledge to disharmonize and to destroy. They were able to provoke heart attacks and other pathological cardiac states with ease.

Once the bases are deactivated and the obsessors gathered, it is still necessary to undo the magnetic fields, which, otherwise, will go on vibrating for an indeterminate time.

You can download Dr Lacerda's book 'Spirit and Matter' from the website of the Holistic Intuition Society:

www.dowsers.ca/SpiritMatter.pdf

Notes

Chapter 5

Baby Souls

Abstracted from 'A Cry from the Womb'
The book written by Gwendolyn Awen Jones
ISBN 9780 974 073 019

Gwendolyn is a medical intuitive and clairvoyant healer who has suffered rape, abortion, and miscarriage. She sees the problems that these cause in a person's aura, and tells how to heal the damage.

Of special interest is her experience in helping many women to be free of attachments of baby souls that cause major problems in their own life, and assisting these baby souls (who were not born or died young) to be healed and get back into 'the light' - a task which we include in our exorcism techniques.

In this book Gwendolyn explains how a soul comes into a fetus, its sensitivity to the emotional and physical environment of the parents, and how influences from relations have a major effect on the future life of a baby throughout its life.

This book is packed with most informative case histories - a 'must read' for all associated with health; many of these demonstrate the failure of religious ceremonies to adequately serve those who need their help.

Gwendolyn has the ability to see each of the metaphysical bodies separated (although they inter-penetrate) and thus examine them in detail to determine the sources of problems.

The Fetus

Gwendolyn's experience is that the Spirit of a child exists independently as a being in its own right before conception occurs; it enters the fetus at conception, and the fetus develops under the influence of the Spirit, the parents, and the environment.

It seems to choose the mother, and perhaps hangs around waiting for a fetus in which to incarnate. The higher levels of Souls may use a more complicated system, where the Spirit of the Soul, mother, and father agree on the incarnation.

The fetus is a conscious being from conception, and prepares for human life by absorbing information from its mother and from what it understands of the attitudes of other people who associate with the mother. In some cases these attitudes may not be correctly understood, but any negativity seems to be taken more seriously than positive influences.

These, especially being 'not wanted' for any reason or by any person, can have extreme repercussions in later life.

The Higher Self

Gwendolyn considers that the Higher Self is Spirit - an aspect of God-Consciousness that is our true nature, 'an individualized essence of God's own Being'. She sees this as a bright light, shining like a star, connected by a golden or silver thread to the soul at a point just above the head.

This light may be overshadowed by events in this or other lives; a dark split in the light may indicate a near death experience, suicide, or intended abortion.

In a healthy person the light appears bright and has a strong connection to the soul. A tenuous link can indicate a weak person or someone with many difficulties.

The Soul

A healthy soul shows as a bright golden ovoid, full of vitality, that extends several feet beyond the physical body. Difficulties in this (or other lives) can show as dark shapes.

These include the effects of dogmatic religious beliefs that can block the natural life force coming from the Higher Self - especially beliefs of guilt and shame.

The effects of the attachments of discarnate Beings at this (and lower levels) can be devastating. These may include deceased family members, the Souls of children who were not born or died young, and Souls from past lives that maintain a close connection - especially if karmic issues are involved.

Damage from recreational drugs, pharmaceuticals, chemotherapy, and radiation can be seen, clouding the Soul or 'shriveling it so it cannot breathe'.

The Mental Body

This body can be very contorted and lose it ovoid shape due to the action of deleterious influences, such as negative thoughts, accidents, and violence; they may become more like spiky black barbed wire than the correct clear radiant lemon-gold translucent egg.

As Gwendolyn brings in light she can see images like watching a movie in full colour; they may be from this or previous lifetimes - even from thousands of years before. Finding and healing the primary cause usually heals the effects in later lifetimes.

The Astral (Dream) Body

This body is very responsive to our thoughts and feelings, and is easily damaged by drugs, alcohol, and general anesthesia - and it can remain damaged for years after surgery, with the person constantly dragging and feeling tired.

A healthy astral body is essential for us to recharge during sleep, and so return home to the Spiritual Realms for education. Failing this dreams may be centered on the lower Astral - the dwelling place of the dead who have not returned into the light.

The astral body can become mis-aligned by a sudden impact, such as a car crash. Physical violence, emotional abuse, or even severe pain can incite the astral body to separate from the physical body.

The Emotional Body

It is through this body that we feel our environment; it should be ovoid, clear, and bright - but can be very damaged from trauma in this and previous lives. In such cases it can look 'like an overstuffed pillow bulging in all directions'. It may even have big black holes in it.

When tired at the emotional level it may show as grey and sluggish, lacking vibrant life force. It can have dirty black-red colours representing old hurts and rage, dirty green with old envies, or filthy yellow with jealousy.

The emotional body may have discarnate entities attached; and when we do not let go of grief, guilt, or other unfinished business when a loved one passes on, we may bind them to us - to our own and their detriment.

The Etheric Body

This is the electrical matrix that includes the meridians used by acupuncturists. It should be a beautiful golden network of light, full of 'chi' life force.

It can be thrown out of alignment or damaged by a heavy fall or blow.

Gwendolyn often finds the energy sacs of deceased Souls from stillbirths, miscarriages, or abortions still attached to the mother. This alone can be a major reason for physical pain in a woman's body - the grief and entanglement can block her etheric flow of life force, causing illness.

Many surgical operations leave the etheric body in a state of chaos - especially epidurals that may cause enormous damage, impeding the flow of life force in the spine.

The Physical Body

Gwendolyn scans the cells in a body for a healthy vibrational sequence - they should have a bright field around them and rotate clockwise - if anti-clockwise, they are diseased. If they are very dim or dark a serious disease, such as cancer, is on its way.

Heavy congestion of the liver can cause the cellular energy to be heavy, slow, and dark red.

She sees healing occurring as colours of different hues, strengths, and vibrations are radiated through the body downwards from the head; many times she sees old dark thought forms and sometimes entities being purged from the physical matrix as this happens.

Thought Forms

These are thoughts that have been energized with emotion - the negative and detrimental ones are often created subconsciously when trauma occurs, and can rule the body without awareness of the conscious mind.

They can be created by the individual alone, in concert with others, or by others acting against the person as in brainwashing, ritual magic, abuse, hexes, and curses.

These have actual shapes and colours - and are 'real things' in the metaphysical world.

For example, you can create a thought form of a barrier to protect you from an assailant, and see the assailant be stopped from attacking you - blocked by the wall (for example) that you have built with your mind, which appears real to the mind of your assailant.

In the same way you can surround yourself with a ball of the intense golden white light of Unconditional True Holy Love to protect you in situations such as healing other people or doing exorcism.

The Inner Child

Gwendolyn considers the Inner Child to be the Spiritual aspect of a person that came into incarnation aware of its Spiritual mission. For vibrant health, it should be in total harmony with the Higher Self, being connected through the Heart centre.

When a person has been thwarted early in life, the Inner Child becomes sad and distant, nothing seems to go right, and life is a mystery - "Why am I here ?" never gets answered.

When she looks at the Inner Child, if the person has gone through trauma, she sees a very young person that is sad or angry, is hiding and no longer in the Heart centre, and with poor flow of life force. Sometimes, if the pregnancy was unwanted, it may not have progressed beyond the fetus stage.

In cases of severe trauma such as family abuse part of the Inner Child may split off and separate - developing a different personality - leading to the recognized multiple personality disorder.

The Chakras

Each of these comprise rotating 'petals' of different numbers and colours. These interpenetrate the bodies of a person, and are connected to the glands (and hence organs) and muscles of the body.

They act rather like microwave dish aerials, bring in information and energy. They should all be rotating clockwise and be free of blockages and interference.

Double Souls

Not mentioned in her book, but discussed with Gwendolyn and other healers, is the case when a discarnate baby Soul hangs around the mother and gets into the next baby to be born.

It is probable that if two souls occupy the same person there will be conflicts. A strong female Soul overriding the correct Soul for a male body will usually produce a 'gay' male - and the reverse a lesbian. If both are the same sex, the maleness (or femaleness) will be extra strong.

In most cases I do not consider it advisable or proper to interfere with the existing situation, unless this is specifically requested, since the person is usually accustomed to the situation and has built a life on that basis.

If the disincarnate baby Soul is immediately taken back into Heaven then this sort of situation would not occur - another reason for all cases of disincarnate baby Souls to be correctly taken into the light whenever needed. The present religious ceremonies do not seem to be sufficient in this regard for those who have been born, and are non-existent for pregnancies that end before birth.

You can download 2 interviews of Gwendolyn Awen Jones by Dr Keith Scott-Mumby from the Holistic Intuition Society's Dowsing website:

www.dowsers.ca/LostChild1.mp3

www.dowsers.ca/LostChild2.mp3

<u>Notes</u>

Chapter 3

I am Sorry.	Please Forgive Me.
I Love you.	Thank You.

The Power of Love

HO'OPONOPONO - by Joe Vitale*

Two years ago, I heard about a therapist in Hawaii who cured a complete ward of criminally insane patients-- without ever seeing any of them. The psychologist would study an inmate's chart and then look within himself to see how he created that person's illness. As he improved himself, the patient improved.

When I first heard this story, I thought it was an urban legend. How could anyone heal anyone else by healing himself? How could even the best self-improvement master cure the criminally insane? It didn't make any sense. It wasn't logical, so I dismissed the story.

However, I heard it again a year later. I heard that the therapist had used a Hawaiian healing process called ho 'oponopono. I had never heard of it, yet I couldn't let it leave my mind. If the story was at all true, I had to know more. I had always understood 'total responsibility' to mean that I am responsible for what I think and do.

Beyond that, it's out of my hands. I think that most people think of total responsibility that way. We're responsible for what we do, not what anyone else does - but that's wrong.

The Hawaiian therapist who healed those mentally ill people would teach me an advanced new perspective about total responsibility. His name is Dr. Ihaleakala Hew Len.

We probably spent an hour talking on our first phone call. I asked him to tell me the complete story of his work as a therapist.

He explained that he worked at Hawaii State Hospital for four years. That ward where they kept the criminally insane was dangerous.

* The 'I' refers to Joe Vitale.

Psychologists quit on a monthly basis. The staff called in sick a lot or simply quit. People would walk through that ward with their backs against the wall, afraid of being attacked by patients. It was not a pleasant place to live, work, or visit.

Dr. Len told me that he never saw patients. He agreed to have an office and to review their files. While he looked at those files, he would work on himself. As he worked on himself, patients began to heal.

"After a few months, patients that had to be shackled were being allowed to walk freely," he told me. "Others who had to be heavily medicated were getting off their medications. And those who had no chance of ever being released were being freed." I was in awe. "Not only that," he went on, "but the staff began to enjoy coming to work".

"Absenteeism and turnover disappeared. We ended up with more staff than we needed because patients were being released, and all the staff was showing up to work. Today, that ward is closed."

This is where I had to ask the million dollar question: "What were you doing within yourself that caused those people to change?"

"I was simply healing the part of me that created them," he said. I didn't understand. Dr. Len explained that total responsibility for your life means that everything in your life - simply because it is in your life, is your responsibility. In a literal sense the entire world is your creation.

Whew. This is tough to swallow. Being responsible for what I say or do is one thing. Being responsible for what everyone in my life says or does is quite another. Yet, the truth is this: if you take complete responsibility for your life, then everything you see, hear, taste, touch, or in any way experience is your responsibility because it is in your life.

This means that terrorist activity, the president, the economy or anything you experience and don't like - is up for you to heal. They don't exist, in a manner of speaking, except as projections from inside you. The problem isn't with them, it's with you, and to change them, you have to change you.

I know this is tough to grasp, let alone accept or actually live. Blame is far easier than total responsibility, but as I spoke with Dr. Len, I began to realize that healing for him and in ho 'oponopono means loving yourself.

If you want to improve your life, you have to heal your life. If you want to cure anyone, even a mentally ill criminal you do it by healing you.

I asked Dr. Len how he went about healing himself. What was he doing, exactly, when he looked at those patients' files?

"I just kept saying, 'I'm sorry' and 'I love you' over and over again," he explained.

"That's it?" - YES

Turns out that loving yourself is the greatest way to improve yourself, and as you improve yourself, you improve your world.

Let me give you a quick example of how this works: one day, someone sent me an email that upset me. In the past I would have handled it by working on my emotional hot buttons or by trying to reason with the person who sent the nasty message.

This time, I decided to try Dr. Len's method. I kept silently saying, "I'm sorry" and "I love you"; I didn't say it to anyone in particular. I was simply evoking the spirit of love to heal within me what was creating the outer circumstance.

Within an hour I got an e-mail from the same person. He apologized for his previous message. Keep in mind that I didn't take any outward action to get that apology. I didn't even write him back. Yet, by saying "I love you", I somehow healed within me what was creating him.

I later attended a ho 'oponopono workshop run by Dr. Len. He's now 70 years old, considered a grandfatherly shaman, and is somewhat reclusive. He praised my book 'The Attractor Factor'. He told me that as I improve myself, my book's vibration will raise, and everyone will feel it when they read it. In short, as I improve, my readers will improve.

"What about the books that are already sold and out there?" I asked. "They aren't out there", he explained, once again blowing my mind with his mystic wisdom. "They are still in you." In short, there is no 'out there'. It would take a whole book to explain this advanced technique with the depth it deserves.

Suffice to say that whenever you want to improve anything in your life, there's only one place to look: inside you. When you look, do it with love.

Synchronicity Strikes Again !

When I was about halfway through the first draft of this book, I felt prompted to go to our monthly Island Fire Hall Book sale.

Once there, my eyes went to a book by Joe Vitale, whose name I recognized from the story on the Hawaiian healing method called Ho'oponopono above.

The book was called 'Zero Limits', published by John Wiley & Sons, ISBN 978-0-470-10147-6, and it told the whole story of Dr Joe Vitale working with the co-author, Dr Ihaleakala Hew Len - the therapist who did the clearing of the mental ward.

When I got home I started to read it - and could not put it down. Finally, at midnight, I went to bed, having read only half of the book - but I could not get to sleep until 3:30 in the morning - my Mind-Brain team was so very excited at the stuff that we had learnt in the book !

Perhaps my Heart, my Mind, my Brain, and my total Being were continually repeating the lessons learnt, and sending Ho'oponopono to all in Creation.

In that sleep I had a most unusual dream - that 'the Bells of Heaven were Ringing, and All in Heaven Singing' - in honour of Morrnah Nalamaku Simeona, the Kahuna for teaching Ihaleakala Hew Len, for him for putting it in practice, and for Joe Vitale who spread the word.

The sub-title of the book is "The Secret Hawaiian System for Wealth, Health, Peace, and More'. In this chapter I will try to explain the major points mentioned in the book concerning health, as seen from my perspective.

This is the sort of book that has a different, but always positive, effect for each person who reads it - being very worthwhile and most beneficial for all.

'We are All the Same'

In my cosmology, we are all composed of tiny cosmic energies working in teams to do different dances, at different speeds, in different planes of existence, to form different higher level Beings to do different jobs.

Ho'oponopono is based on a similar principle - that we are 'All the Same', in a holographic universe of some description.

In Ho'oponopono we go one step further - we recognize that we, ourselves, are intimately involved in everything that happens, that we can take responsibility for it, and that we can do something about it by working on ourselves - since we are all part of the holograph.

This works because in a holograph every part contains the whole of the holograph. So we contain all the problems that everyone bears - and by healing that part in ourselves we heal that same part in others.

I suggest that all healers incorporate Ho'oponopono in the modalities that they use. In each session of therapy define Ho'oponopono for themselves:

> **We are all the same - all part of 'The One'.**
> **I accept responsibility for all that occurs.**
> **I am Sorry.**   **Please Forgive Me.**
> **I Love you.**   **Thank You.**

Then keep repeating 'Ho'oponopono' to themselves whilst doing the therapy. Remember that Love is the strongest power in all creation - Love that is non-judgmental, without restriction. I call this 'True Holy Love, Namaste'.

I suggest that we add lines to the basic statement to acknowledge that we are all the same, and that we take responsibility. I believe that these additions reinforce the acceptance by our sub-conscious and improve the healing ability.

This would be an excellent way of keeping the logical mind-brain occupied - getting it out of the way. Perhaps a connection to the morphic field of Ho'oponopono would also be beneficial.

I am doing this procedure with my exorcism work - using a Pendulum over the picture of the person involved, so as to magnify the thoughts that are sent by Ho'oponopono to all concerned with that person.

I rotate my Pendulum clockwise to do this - then it starts to make 'waves', indicating that the Angelic Beings are at work. Finally it stops, showing that work is completed for the moment. I repeat this every few days for each person, more frequently for those in great need.

There are many modalities for creating one's own reality, including healing - some work better than others for certain people in various circumstances; most do not work perfectly in every case.

A common factor in most is that we think that we are doing the work. When we do it ourselves we do so within the limits imposed by ourselves. Miracles happen when we get out of the way - and let them occur with zero limits. When we stop thinking that we are in charge, and know that we are just doing our part as guided by our intuition.

Memory Blockages

Most of the blocks to success are held in our memories, which are always accessed by our sub-conscious before any conscious thought arises or action occurs.

These blocks are like programs, one aspect leading to another. It seems that the priority is in accordance with the emotions attached.

EFT is one way of dissolving these emotions, so that although we may still have the memory there is little importance attached to it - so that it no longer affects our lives.

Using Ho'oponopono is another way - and has the advantage that we do not need to consciously link to the emotions involved. Thus when we continually use Ho'oponopono on ourselves we do 'spring cleaning' on all our memories and our sub-conscious.

Dr Hew Len tells "If you have a challenge with somebody, it is not with that person! It is that memory that is coming up that you are reacting to. That is what you have a challenge with. It is not the other person". Perhaps due to the emotional entanglement of that memory!

We do not have to know the cause of a pain or a problem - just apply Ho'oponopono to it, or where it appears to be.

Some healers suggest that we place unwanted things on our clipboard, as in computer technology. Dr Hew Len points out that although this puts this out of sight, it is still in your computer; you need to empty the recycle bin to remove it completely. Even then, it may still be in your 'back-up'. Perhaps it is best to 'clean' our memories with Ho'oponopono, rather than remove them or clear them away.

Zero State

Joe Vitale suggests that we return to the "zero state where there are no thoughts, words, deeds, memories, programs, beliefs, or anything else. Just nothing. Where nothing exists - but everything is possible".

You may share my belief that this is beyond the ability of most of us - certainly on a full-time basis. But perhaps that is the condition that we reach when we go into our 'Heart Space'.

I am also not sure that we should completely relinquish our 'free will'. I do know that we must keep an 'open mind' - and especially be fully open to our intuition, our inspiration, at all times.

Dr Hew Len tells "What we individually hold, memories or inspiration, have an immediate and absolute impact on everything from humanity to the mineral, vegetable, and animal kingdom" - as do all the changes made. Perhaps he should have added "all the Spiritual planes, all the associated morphic fields".

He adds "The purpose of life is to be restored back to Love, moment to moment. To fulfill this purpose, the individual must acknowledge that he is 100 per cent responsible for creating his life the way it is. He must come to see that it is his thoughts that create his life the way it is from moment to moment. The problems are not people, places, and situations, but rather the thoughts of them. He must come to appreciate that there is no such place as 'out there'."

The Power of Love

This is a picture of David before an exorcism.

A young child attachment shows in his head - due to some trauma that happened when he was about 5 years old, together with a Soul fragment and thought forms probably from a family member that died.

Around the shoulder is a Soul Program that is blocking his heart in this life.

Attachments around his hip and leg are recognized as astral fragments from other soldiers that died during fights.

Other dark shadows indicate further problems that need to be healed, having various causes.

In the 'after' picture (not shown) the darkness has all been cleared away - due to the healing given by exorcism !

This exorcism was performed by Kaye Jensen who is a most experienced clairvoyant Healer - and one of the best adjusters of the Assemblage Beam which controls our behaviour throughout life.

The images show here were obtained via an 'Indigo Qx' artificial intelligence machine, designed by Dr Bill Nelson who worked at NASA, and used mainly for stress management.

The colour of David's aura changed to be the pink colour of unconditional love.

Kaye tells how she was guided to 'inject unconditional Love' into David, which she did in her imagination.

This is similar to the pouring in of Love recommended by the late Harold McCoy of the Ozark Research Institute.

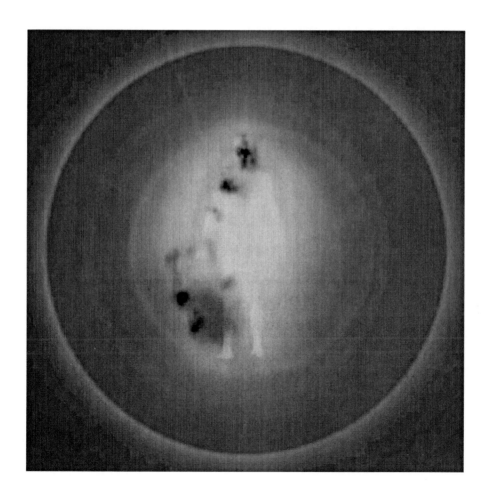

'True Holy Love, Namaste' is like the unconditional love of a parent - "I love you, but I do not like bad behaviour - I ask you to change your behaviour to be good, and I will help you as best I can".

Ho'oponopono

We are all the same

- all part of 'The One'.

I accept responsibility for all that occurs.

I am Sorry.   Please Forgive Me.

I Love you.   Thank You.

Chapter 7

The Basis of Holistic Exorcism

All this long distance exorcism is done by the Angelic Beings; the part played by the exorcist is to connect Heart to Heart to communicate with the person being exorcised, to note the problems identified and determine their severity, to send energy from the exorcist to the Angelic Beings that they can use in the exorcism, and to record changes made.

Further healing may be needed, such as clearing the aura, using Emotional Freedom Techniques (EFT), time/space travel, Reiki, and manually extracting entities as directed.

The exorcist uses a check list, as included later in this book, first to record the original conditions found, second to link with the needed healing, and third to record the changes that are understood to have been accomplished. The same record for the person is used in repeated sessions that check current conditions and indicate any further exorcism that is needed.

At the completion of each session an overall clean-up is given, protection is placed, more energy sent to the Angelic Beings, and gratitude with love is sent to all who helped in the exorcism and healing.

Healing is needed not only for the person being exorcised, but also for those entities that were causing the problems, so that they are free of all needs to hurt any being. This is far superior to 'sending them to the ends of the universe' as practiced by inferior exorcists.

All this work is done by the Angelic Beings, a catch-all term for members of the 'Force for Good' in the non-physical realms, and which includes departed souls, Angels, Arch Angels, and Beings at even higher levels.

Since the dark forces infest all combinations of communities and religions, we do not rely on any one 'Divine Being'.

In this regard it is probable that the all the Angelic Being have specific skills and abilities - and help comes best from them when they work together in a co-ordinated team, with each member contributing according to their own abilities.

One way of working with such teams is to access 'The System' as taught by the late Walter Woods. Using your Pendulum (rotating clockwise) over your 'Handy Chart' (explained later) open in 'True Holy Love' to 'The System', explain what is needed, and ask if 'The System' is willing and able to ensure that the task is correctly completed. Your Pendulum will start to swing over '10' if 'The System' will so assist, and then start to make swings from '0' through to '10' as each aspect of the problem is healed. When it stays swinging over '10' all of the task that can be healed at this time is completed. It is best to now ask if anymore work is needed, and whether it can be done at this time.

Experience has shown that this 'Good God System' knows the skills and abilities of helpers and co-ordinates their endeavors to get the needed results. This is covered in the 'Preparing for Exorcism' procedure.

Dark forces may be attached to the Healee - and also to the Souls, etc. that are attached to or associated with the Healee; these need to be found and traced to their castles and dungeons, and leads (black, grey cords) followed to any higher commanders in the dark forces - and to any leads from these to other dark groups.

It is understood that clairvoyants and the Angelic Beings sometimes have great difficulty in seeing or finding these cords, and in tracing them to those who control.

It has been found that the Souls of some non-human Beings are of great help in doing this work, so leading the 'Force for Good' to where they can take the needed actions.

These teams of discarnate other Beings will be brought in to action by the Angelic Beings as needed - so you do not have to do anything.

Usually those entrapped in the dungeons can be Healed in the Healing Globes and Spirit Hospitals - or else dealt with so that they will not be able to cause problems in the future.

The higher levels above Souls may also be attacked - so dark force attachments must be investigated in these cases as well and then healed if found. Failure to clear the higher levels may cause the unwanted effects to be re-instated later, thus spoiling the Healing being given.

Working with Heart

The magnetic field from our Hearts is far stronger than that from the brain; our Hearts have their own neurons, command the sub-conscious, and are our link to the Angelic Beings with whom we must co-operate.

One way to 'get into Heart Space' is to place your awareness into your Heart - then to 'speak' (send your thoughts) to your Heart as if it were a separate Being. You may find that in this mode you become non-judgmental, and perhaps your knees may 'soften' so that you bend slightly.

When an application is received, ask your own Heart to connect to the Heart of the person that needs exorcism, and obtain the data required - including information from the healee's sub-conscious. Such a connection is made by a cord of 'Love Light' (Unconditional Love) between the Hearts.

In case that the other Heart has been hurt, it is best to send a clone of your Heart to watch over the person and report back with information.

This sounds weird, but it is easy to accomplish - just ask your Heart, as if it were a separate being, to form a clone and to send it as an observer that reports back to your own Heart, which keeps these reports in memory until needed.

Some people consider that working direct with your Heart is best because it by-passes ego. But it is preferable to realize that the ego has an important task - to manipulate data. Thus the superior way is to get your ego working as a good team member under the leadership of your Heart - no energy wasted in in-fighting, but a combined effort for good.

It is important that all these communications are between your Heart (not your conscious self) and the Heart of the Healee or the consciousness of the fragment or actual Soul / Spirit involved - especially any dark entities or those infested by them.

This is to help prevent any such entity from trying to attach itself to you or trying to possess you. Your Heart will use your memory to store needed information.

Dowsing - Signals from your Intuition

When you ask your Heart a question that should yield a simple YES or NO answer, your Heart-Mind-Brain team can manipulate your nervous-muscular system to give a signal.

The simplest way is to stand up straight, ask your Heart to signal YES by swaying you forward (or backwards for NO), and then ask your Heart "Is this signal understood and accepted?" - your body should sway forward. If not immediately successful, keep on until you do get success.

Another and easier signal is to define a movement of your tongue - YES indicated by your tongue touching the roof of your mouth, NO by it dropping to your jaw. This is very quick, and unobservable to other people.

Practicing these will give you a simple and effective tool that can help you in many ways in various aspects of your life.

These body signals only indicate YES or NO - so more signals are needed to select from choices; a Pendulum such as a bead on a string can point to selections on a chart.

There are two signaling systems with a Pendulum. The physical system is 'to and fro' for YES (symbolizing a joining, such as "Is this food good for me to eat?") and 'side to side' for NO, symbolizing a barrier.

The metaphysical system is best used in all healing work - a clockwise rotation (the way that good energies move in a spiral) indicating YES and sending Love and healing, anti-clockwise for NO and to extract 'not good' energies.

One aspect of sending Love and healing with a Pendulum is unknown by many experienced Dowsers. When you rotate your Pendulum clockwise, the string and bead forms a cone shape (a circular pyramid) similar to the paper cone that magnifies sound in a loud speaker.

This magnifies the thoughts that you send thousands of times, so that Love and healing that you send is much more powerful and effective.

Remember that what you send to others comes back to you - so never send out any bad or hurtful thoughts !

Using a Ptah Pendulum is even more effective, since energies are very reactive to shape.

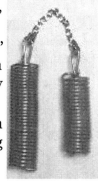

The Ptah Pendulum extracts 'not good' energies, heals them in the long coil, then sends them up to the short coil where they are polished and sent out as Love.

For full details on the use of a Ptah Pendulum see our main web page and click on 'Dowsing & Healing Tools' in the Service Category.

Overall Explanations

Implants such as poisoned objects and (electro-)chemical/ mechanical devices may have been implanted, sometimes with 'Booby Traps' to prevent removal or to install replacements. A most careful search must be made for these, for any associated booby-traps, and for any 'maintenance workers'. These must be identified and completely de-activated.

A Life Mission usually is given to and accepted by an incarnating Soul. A great clairvoyant healer, Kaye Jansen, who specializes in Assemblage work, discovered that in some cases the Life Mission was given by the dark forces disguised as Beings of Light.

This is believed to be rare, but should be checked - and if so, the Life Mission canceled and replaced with one of Love. Kaye's website is http://www.clearyourpath.ca

Forgiveness is important since if the healee is holding onto emotions such as anger, hate, or jealousy dark forces will continue to be attracted. See Appendix A.

"I forgive all who hurt me, and I ask forgiveness from all I hurt. I forgive myself for all mistakes made with good intent. I understand that this forgiveness shall be so providing my intent is to stay 'In the Light' of the 'Good God Energy' for all eternities"

The Hi Aukamura are understood to be Beings in charge of Soul Groups in universes, the Aukamura control Soul Groups in galaxies, with Higher Selves commanding Soul Groups in the various earths - and their associated Heavens.

Aukamura is a Huna term having a meaning similar to Higher Self, used here to differentiate between the levels involved.

It is important to check on their values from the top down, since if they have been hurt (including possession by fragments or similar) this has repercussions on all that they control.

Failure to Heal these Beings will probably allow the hurts and problems being Healed to be re-manifested in the Healee.

By sending them Healing in cases where they have been hurt, you are likely to help all under their jurisdiction - so having a Healing effect on others in this earth, in this galaxy, and in this universe, etc.

We check for their value, if darkness is attached, and if they have been hurt - so that the needed help may be sent to them by the Angelic Beings.

Soul Spirits should be checked for number (in case of intrusion) and their values, and if dark forces are attached. First the dark forces are cleared, and then intrusive Souls removed (if advisable - see comments in the chapter about Baby Souls) and sent to their correct place.

Past Life influences may be having a detrimental effect on the Higher Self, in all the Soul Group, and for this particular Soul.   This includes retribution from those that they have hurt in previous existences.

In this context the previous action by one member of the Soul Group may result in attacks on another of the group, due to similarities in their Being. Again we check for the numbers involved and their values.

The Assemblage Beam is not strictly part of exorcism but it has a major influence on a person's personality and behaviour, and if not corrected may prevent any improvement.

The point of entry should be centered, and the angle of the beam should be at right angles to the body. Usually the centre is slightly higher in females (they are often more emotional) than in males.   These are marked 'F' and 'M' on the diagram shown on the next page.

The beam itself, about 2 yards or 2 metres in length, must be straight, without bends, kinks, or twists, and should be of equal lengths back and front of the body. Entry below 'The Gap' indicates approaching death.

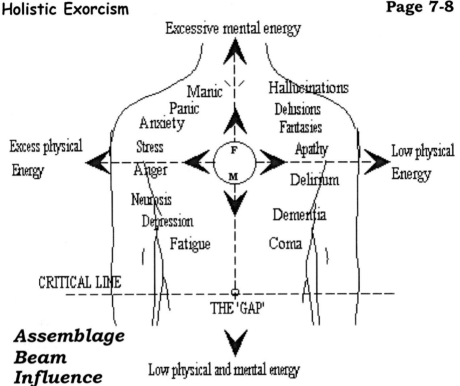

Excessive mental energy

Manic
Panic
Anxiety
Stress
Anger
Neurosis
Depression
Fatigue

Hallucinations
Delusions
Fantasies
Apathy
Delirium
Dementia
Coma

Excess physical Energy

Low physical Energy

CRITICAL LINE

THE 'GAP'

Assemblage Beam Influence

Low physical and mental energy

The first person to publicize the Assemblage Point was Dr Jonathan Whale - in his excellent book 'The Catalyst of Power'; website: www.whalemedical.com/ap1.html

Energy suckers may be draining the life essence from the healee. These may be astral vampires or other human beings.

The Guardian Angel of the Healee cannot be assumed to be perfect, although this is desirable. Sometimes they have been hurt themselves, or are just not worthy. So we check on their condition and their value, and get any needed change made.

The Akashic Record and Karma of the Healee is checked; in many cases the 'not good' incidents have been caused by the interference by dark forces in previous lives - and so should not be counted against the Karma of the Healee. In such cases the Lords of Karma are petitioned to revise the Akashic Record and Karma of the Healee.

The Super-consciousness, consciousness, and the sub-conscious of the Healee may have intrusions. In each case we check the number in the Healee and their values, and if dark forces are attached.

It is useful to check if the sub-conscious is causing hurts to the Healee in a misguided attempt to protect - this is typical of allergies, due to some hurt happening at a certain time and becoming associated wrongly with a particular substance.

Guides are investigated in the same way. Some seem to be acting in their own interest, and not in the best interest of the Healee. If so, they must be removed and replaced with good guides.

The Heart team needs to always operate in True Holy Love, Namaste, and the ego and sub-conscious must be willing to work under the leadership of the Heart.

We check for the value of the Heart and for any damage that has occurred.

Other Entities may be around the home or workplace and cause problems - an example would be a deceased resident who has not passed on but is stuck in the earth plane.

These need to be identified and action taken to heal them and take them to their correct place.

Other Energies are similar - these may be hexes or curses put on the land, the home, the family, or the Healee. If a person sleeps or sits in a noxious earth or electro-magnetic energy field then their health may suffer - these are not subject to exorcism, but need blessing to help them become beneficial.

Negative Programs may have been beneficial when a young child, but are now inappropriate; do they still exist and operate ?

These include statements and orders heard which have been taken 'as gospel'. They also include non-beneficial beliefs that have a negative impact on the Healee.

<u>Fragments of Souls</u> are a major source of problems. These may come from other Souls including babies who were not born or died young, from animals, be extra-terrestrial, or of the Healee's own Soul - due to serious abuse or trauma, resulting in a split to provide protection of the Being. It is best to check for dark forces that are attached to fragments.

In most cases these splits of the Healee's own Soul will respond favourably to love and assurances that (since circumstances have changed) it is now safe for them to return.

It is important that the 'film in the mind' of the occurrence that originated the fragment be changed to one that is beneficial and accepted by the fragment, which in this state has its own existence in the matrix.

In rare cases, especially when a fragment has gained experience of separate and domineering control, they may prove very resistant.

This may be most likely to happen when the Healee has been an amoral, dominating controller in a past life - and the value obtained is in the 4 to 6 range.

In very rare cases the fragment may have gained special abilities due to witchcraft activities or from previous incarnations; if these are being used in a non-benevolent manner these powers and skills must be removed.

<u>Other Non-Beneficial Interference</u> may be present - this is a 'catch all' just in case something has been missed.

<u>Other Negative Influences</u> should be checked to identify their type, values, and sources. At this point we can recheck if there are any more past life problems that still need action to be taken.

if <u>Apometrics</u> is needed, then the Astral body of the healee will be taken to a Spirit Hospital and all the necessary work done during sleep time. It is now understood that a medium is not required.

This includes all needed work on the Assemblage Beam, which controls all Chakras, glands, and organs, as well as removing all unwanted influences in all the auras - which have a major effect on the etheric body and hence the physical body.

Since this work is so extensive, it may be that Apometrics is all that will be needed in the future to ensure good health.

Other Healing Modalities

Bill Ellis, in his book 'Vibrational Energy Healing' (published by the Holistic Intuition Society), suggests that clearing and energizing the Chakras is needed in most Healing work. In the 'Distant Healing Manual' are facsimiles of Touch Stones (linked energetically to the actual stones) with diagrams of both the 7 major Chakras and the those in the Pranic Triangle. The charts for Chakras are included. You can print these and use them in your Healing work. The actual Touch Stones are not being made now.

The 'Distant Healing Manual' is a FREE download from our website http://www.in2it.ca (go to 'Healing Overview' - download instructions are at the bottom of that page.

'Hands On' Healing

I use a teddy bear to represent a male, and a doll as a token for a female; I place a paper with the name, location, and birth date on the token and ask that the token now represent the person.

Presuming that the answer is YES, I then use my Ptah Pendulum to work on their aura, putting love where needed, removing unwanted energy, and always ending by putting in more love.

When you link your Heart to the Heart of the healee, your Heart is aware of all the problems - so you can ask your Heart to guide you where your hands should be placed on (or near) the Doll or Teddy to act as a conduit for healing or to pull out 'bad energies'.

My Heart places my hands wherever they are needed and uses them to take any action that is required - my hands become the tools of the Angelic Beings who are doing the healing.

This may just be connecting to places where the energy needs to be changed, or pulling out (with my etheric hands!) stuff that needs to be removed and sent for further healing - including to use the technique developed by Harold McCoy (past President of the American Society of Dowsers and founder of the Ozark Research Institute - for Metaphysical Healing).

His suggestions include unzipping the top of a token's head, using a hose to pour in love energy, a vacuum hose to extract whatever is causing problems (often my hands being guided to pull out bad stuff) and then finishing by pouring more love into the head and zipping it back again.

Radionics is a method of determining the frequency of a health problem and then sending another frequency which cancels the one that is causing the problem.

More than one problem may need attention, so imagining that you are playing an organ can make a far more complete vibrational pattern which you send to the Healee.

EFT (Emotional Freedom Technique) is a system developed by Gary Craig of tapping into your meridians and sub-conscious to identify and heal problems. This has been extended by Karl Dawson into 'Matrix ReImprinting' to include tapping on the energy beings involved and making beneficial changes to the remembered incidents.

Karl's major contribution is to ensure that these changes are recorded in the Matrix / Akashic Records, so that they benefit all who were involved in the incidents, thus reducing any bad karma.

Timelines are useful in getting to the origin of problems. This is similar to the 'German New Medicine' approach, which indicates that all problems followed some sort of trauma - and that what are perceived as symptoms may well be the cure in progress.

Time travel may be used to clear memories of traumatic events - taking the conscious and sub-conscious back in time to before whatever happened and then bringing them back without exposure to the happening.

This can be done using EFT (Gary Craig's Emotional Freedom Techniques) especially the extension developed by Karl Dawson (MatrixReimprinting.com) or by the methods taught by Dr Richard Bartlett.

The work of Karl Dawson is exceptionally good - it is his brilliant understanding of the treatment needed to heal the personal fragments / inner child (which he calls 'ECHOs' - Energy Conscious Holograms) that leads us to change the actual visual scenes held in the matrix.

If memories are not held only in our cells or auras, but have links to the actual memories in the Matrix, the Fields, or the Akashic Records, (probably all the same) then changing the remembered circumstances for a more beneficial outcome may make the change for all who were involved, including any Karmic implications.

Samuel Sagan, MD, has found that many intrusive life forms, including fragments from deceased Souls and from other dimensions) hide in the muscular structures of humans and may be the cause of 'pains that move'.

Notes

Chapter 8

Exorcism at Work

When a request for exorcism is received use your Pendulum over the personal details until it ceases to swing, and repeat this for the problems listed; now ask your Heart to send a clone of your Heart to the Healee to observe and report on the situation.

Print the pages to be used for healing, complete the identity information, and attach to application.

Check with your Heart for advice on when to proceed - usually after the Heart Clone has observed the person for a few days.

Preparation

First of all go to the 'Preparing for Exorcism' page 8-3 and read the overall instructions to your sub-conscious and other systems - so that the directions are all clear and precise.

After you have done this for about 10 times, so that it is well absorbed by you, you may use your Pendulum over these pages to see if they are accepted by all concerned - if a NO swing is given, then re-read these pages to reinforce their acceptance.

Then use your Pendulum to check your present Dowsing Abilities using the special chart on page 8-8.

<u>Do this for each Healee in case of problem at Soul Group or Higher</u>.

Should there be a problem identified, ask your Heart and 'The System' to correct the problem, and then re-check.

Only proceed when you have been signaled GOOD.

Next use your Pendulum over the application sent by the Healee, and check that you have a good connection to the correct person. If there is any problem, ask your Heart to indicate what action should be taken, and check that this is done before proceeding.

The Exorcism

First go through the pages to be used using your Pendulum with the counting charts and your Handy Chart to record the current situation prior to this exorcism.

Repeat - but this time use your Pendulum to make corrections for each item that needs this work - always working from the highest level downwards. <u>As you work on each entry use your Handy Chart to watch any needed corrections being made, such as the removal of intrusive energies for them to be taken for Healing and be in their rightful place.</u>

Go through the check lists again, and record on the sheet the new situation after this exorcism.

After a week or so, check the results (never do this the same day, since you mind may still thinking of the values then obtained and so prejudice your Dowsing).

Completion

To finish go to page 8-11 and follow the instructions 'On Completion of Work for a Healee' - this is when the major portion of your work is manifested, so use you 'Handy Chart' to monitor the progress of the Angelic Beings and 'The System' in doing the exorcism.

Character Overview

The basis for a character overview of the person is outlined on page 8-19 - denoted by percentages of the characteristics that are indicate by your Pendulum using the counting chart (page 8-9). You can form an overall appreciation of the person using this and the records obtained on the previous pages - <u>useful in accessing suitability for a particular job</u> (without exorcism ?) or advising on work needed for personal growth.

Preparing for Exorcism

Read the following and load it into your sub-conscious and other systems:

"I open in True Holy Love, Namaste, and that Love of Truth as a conduit for Healing; I ask that 'The System', 'The Love Namaste Healing Team', and all the Angelic Beings and Healing Energies give their full co-operation and help in this Healing and that all such Healing is done with Unconditional True Holy Love, Namaste, in the way that is best for all concerned without harm or hurt to any. I fill and surround my total Being with the brilliant golden white light of unconditional Love."

"I ask my Heart to make all communications with the Angelic Beings and others in the Healing team, the total Being of the Healee, and all others involved in this exorcism."

"Nothing comes to me which is not mine; nothing goes to others which is not theirs; always excepting Healing given with True Holy Love, Namaste. I remain perfectly protected and grounded in every way. As I help to Heal others, I get Healed myself".

"When using my Pendulum a clockwise rotation shall input Blessing 995 and 885, Healing 997 and 887, and the Healing Energies, Essences, and Vibrational Patterns needed, and transmute all that is dark or non-beneficial to be Light and beneficial; a counter-clockwise rotation shall extract all those that are unwanted or non-beneficial and send them to be Healed with True Holy Love, Namaste in the way that is best for all creation."

"All information given to me shall be the truth, the whole truth, and nothing but the truth - in the way that I can understand using the best of my abilities; if this is not possible, a NOT AVAILABLE signal shall be given. Any failure for me to understand or believe any aspect of the Healings shall not impede the Healings given to the Healee."

"I send my Love, Thanks, and Gratitude, with True Holy Love, Namaste, to All who Help in this Healing and all other Healings in which I participate."

Sending True Holy Love, Namaste to those that are in the darkness is a magnificent way to help them - most have not had any Love sent to them for a very long time - perhaps never !

Initially they may not like this, because it is so different from their usual situation; in such cases send them more Unconditional Love (True Holy Love, Namaste) with Blessing 995 and 885, and Healing 997 and 887, to help them adjust to the Light.

Heart to Heart Communications - <u>read and retain in your sub-conscious memory</u>

It is important that all these communications are between your Heart (not your conscious self) and the Heart of the Healee or the consciousness of the fragment or actual Soul /Spirit involved - especially any dark entities or those infested by them. This is to help prevent any such entity from trying to attach itself to you or trying to possess you.

These are suggestions for your Heart and the Angelic Beings and others that are working in the Healing team to consider and use if appropriate.

- Send True Holy Love, Namaste to the person and to all that are attached and/or possessing.
- Locate any and all darkness in or around the person (i.e. in their aura).
- Go back in time to locate, identify, and nullify the sources of all infestations.
- Locate all dark cords connected to the darkness and trace to other dark entities.
- Communicate with all the commanders of darkness, up to the highest.
- Repeat this for all dark cords from all dark entities until all are in the Light.

- Form a bubble of Light around each darkness in or around the person, send True Holy Love, Namaste and ask :
* Does it have a shape, if so what shape ? Ditto colour, smell.
* What is its intent ?
* What is it trying to do ?
* Was it given a job ? If so, was this job given by those that are 'In the Light' ?
* What does it want for itself ?
* Would it like to be free of all hurts, pains, and suffering ?
* Would it like to be happy and joyful all the time ?
* Was it 'In the Light' at any time before ?
* Go back in time to when 'In the Light', when first formed ?
* How does this feel ?
* Do you want to keep feeling good, to be in the Light in all eternities ?
* Would it like this to happen now ?   If YES, let it be so.
* Charge them to operate with Heart at all times, in all planes, in all dimensions.

If there is resistance, communicate with all the life forms, elementals, etc in the entity, send True Holy Love, Namaste and ask them "Do you like to Hurt, or Love to Heal ?", working with them to help each one to be in the Light, and so dismantle the entity - then the refusing part (elemental Being, etc) loses its strength, can be handled easily. They may be extra-terrestrial, and/or operating in different dimensions.

Search for any hells or pits which may be used to hurt dark entities for whatever reason, and for any 'dead blobs' of darkness, so that all the life forms in these can be healed and be in the Light. Again check for all commanders and all others involved in darkness and heal them and all in them. Bless any shields to be brilliant white light of Good God energy.

Continue this approach seeking all dark cords going from commanders and their minions to those that they control.

Cut all chords and remove all hooks, sending them to be healed.

DECEASED SOULS (now free of darkness)

Locate, send True Holy Love, Namaste and then recognize them by asking:

- Who are you ?
- Are you related in this present life ? In a past life ?
- When did you join or attach to this person ?
- What is your intent ? What are you trying to do ?
- What do you want for yourself ?
- Do you want to be free of all hurts, pains, and suffering ?
- Do you want to be happy and joyful all the time ?
- Do you want to be with its family, friends, in Heaven ?
- Look upwards - can you see Light ? Even a tiny spot ?
- Can you see Angelic Beings or friends or relations nearby ?
- Go now and join with them, in the Light.
- If any problem, may be dark entity - to be healed as above.

FRAGMENTS TO BE RETURNED AND REJOINED

These may have been afraid to return due to a dark entity or a soul attachment that caused them to leave - these should have been healed already; if any are still there then heal as outlined above. Each fragment has a silver cord that still connects to their being.

Fragments of others that have attached to be returned to their own being; those of the person to rejoin in the present now.

Send True Holy Love, Namaste to the fragment, and ask:

- Do you have a name ? (may not if not born, etc.)
- Who did you fragment from ?
- When did you join or attach to this person ?
- What is your intent ? What are you trying to do ?
- What do you want for yourself ?
- Do you want to be free of all hurts, pains, and suffering ?
- Do you want to be happy and joyful all the time ?
- If from another person: (dead or alive) (may be a thought form)
- *   Go now and rejoin that person with True Holy Love, Namaste.
- *   If problem, do healing on that person, or send directly into the Light.

- Do you now know that your person has been healed and is free of the old problems ?
- Can you now trust the person (as a grown-up) ?
- Now rejoin your person in True Holy Love, Namaste.

IMPLANTS - a careful search must be made for poisoned objects and electro/chemical/mechanical devices which may have been implanted, including any associated booby-traps. These must be identified, removed, and de-activated, and any 'maintenance workers' taken to be healed.

It is important to record any changed circumstances in the Matrix/Akashic Record.

Preparing to Dowse

Use the chart on the next page to check your present Dowsing abilities.

Only proceed when you have been signaled GOOD.

Should there be a problem identified, ask your Heart and 'The System' to correct the problem, and then re-check. Use your 'Handy Chart' to monitor the corrections made by 'The System' - when your Pendulum goes to 10 and then stops, ask if any more correction is needed.

When you start work on the check lists / work charts (pages 8-13 to 8-16) first go through the items noting for each one if any problems exist (Y or N or 0 - or numbers found) and their severity (-6 to +6).

Next start again and go through all the items, but this time use your Pendulum and Handy Chart to give energy for healing and check on the action.

When completed, go through all the items again noting all changes made as a result of the work done.

Preparing to Dowse

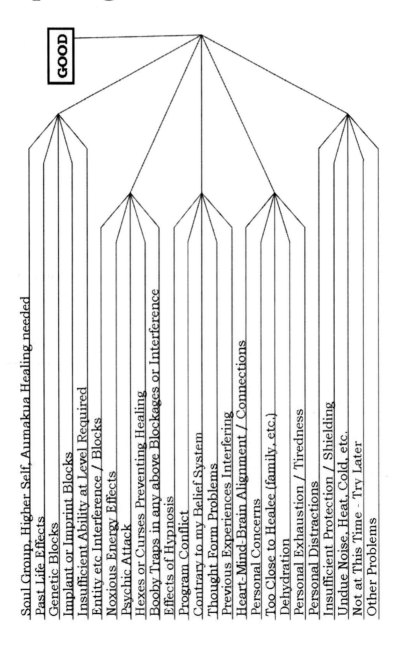

GOOD

Soul Group, Higher Self, Aumakua Healing needed
Past Life Effects
Genetic Blocks
Implant or Imprint Blocks
Insufficient Ability at Level Required
Entity etc Interference / Blocks
Noxious Energy Effects
Psychic Attack
Hexes or Curses Preventing Healing
Booby Traps in any above Blockages or Interference
Effects of Hypnosis
Program Conflict
Contrary to my Belief System
Thought Form Problems
Previous Experiences Interfering
Heart-Mind-Brain Alignment / Connections
Personal Concerns
Too Close to Healee (family, etc.)
Dehydration
Personal Exhaustion / Tiredness
Personal Distractions
Insufficient Protection / Shielding
Undue Noise, Heat, Cold, etc.
Not at This Time – Try Later
Other Problems

Your Handy Chart

Since most of us have two hands, we can use the spare one (the one not holding your Pendulum !) as a chart for many purposes.

It is best to use signals that conform to indicators that you see often, such as the speedometer and charging gauge of your car - your mind-brain team is accustomed to the signals used.

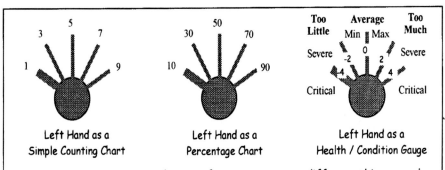

| Left Hand as a Simple Counting Chart | Left Hand as a Percentage Chart | Left Hand as a Health / Condition Gauge |

You can use your ingenuity to let your fingers mean many different things - so long as you have ensured that your Mind-Brain team understands the meanings to be signalled for each 'hand-chart' - and that you have specified to your Mind-Brain team which 'hand-chart' is being used for the Dowsing you are now doing !

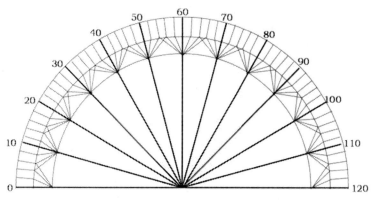

Percentage and Counting Chart

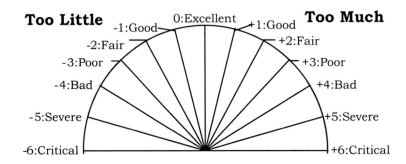

Intensity Chart: The values indicate the following types of problems:

- -6 Mass murderer - will kill for love of killing, without reason; no moral dissuasion.
- -5 Highly dangerous - kill with slightest provocation and little reason.
- -4 Dangerous criminal - murder with provocation or when under duress.
- -3 Character: car thefts, robberies. Abuse / beat family members.
- -2 Basically dishonest - shoplifter or petty thief.
- -1 Little concern for others or for truthfulness; outstanding car salesman or politician !
- 0 is the neutral / balanced mind without problems. <u>Most desirable.</u>
- +1 Broad thinking and stability; highly qualified teacher or counselor.
- +2 Great wisdom, sound metaphysical thinking. Attributes of a mystic.
- +3 Firm in ideals and ideas; typical evangelist.
- +4 Intolerant, inflexible in ideas; minister determined to reform congregation.
- +5 Stubborn in thought, unrelenting, unforgiving; the 'Hanging Judge'.
- +6 Crusader; 'Kill, it is God's Will'.

Time Lines

These charts can be used to find when the cause of a problem occurred. Finding the time of the most recent cause enables that cause to be identified. Finding the 'First Cause' will assist in eliminating the foundation so that subsequent causes will be collapsed.

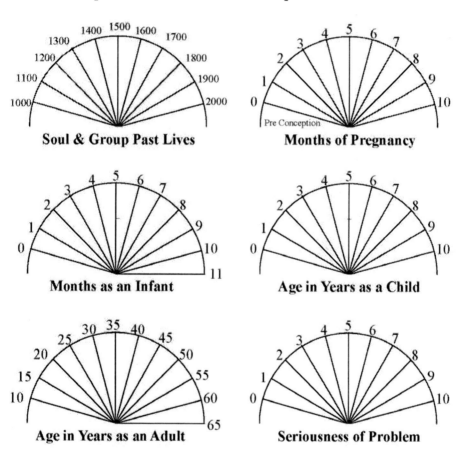

Soul & Group Past Lives

Months of Pregnancy

Months as an Infant

Age in Years as a Child

Age in Years as an Adult

Seriousness of Problem

On Completion of Work for a Healee

Take four deep breathes, exhaling 'HA !' (this is a Huna technique - see note on page 8-21) with the intent to send the energy of these breathes to assist the work being done, and state:

"Let all that are removed be taken to be Healed with True Holy Love, Namaste, in the way that is Best for All and be in their Rightful Place; go now, in Peace, Harmony, and Holy Love, Namaste, to be Healed.

Let Healing Globes and the Love Light of Unconditional Love, True Holy Love, Namaste and all needed vibrational patterns now be placed around and inter-penetrating the Healee and all associated with the Healee, to be fully active in all times and all nows:

- *To Heal, to transmute, and to transform all darkness and all that is non-beneficial (including all memories) into being Light and beneficial.*

- *To protect and operate with True Holy Love, Namaste, with Harmony, and with Peace in all ways and all aspects.*

- *To be completely effective in all planes and all dimensions, all times and all nows."*

Now use your Handy Chart to monitor the Healing being given - your Pendulum will circle clockwise during this process, sometimes pointing at various fingers as individual aspects or entities are Healed.

When completed your Pendulum will point to 10 and not move.

Check by asking "Is any more work needed now ?" and if at this time your Pendulum may make another session as above; again ask at the end, then ask "Is any more work needed in the future ?" and if so, ask "can this work be done automatically when so needed ?" and if NO, ask when, and if you should be involved. If so, this is a commitment to do such work - ask if your Heart can do this on your behalf. If NO then ask to be properly reminded and assisted when your actions are needed.

<u>Then give Thanks:</u>

"I send my Love, Thanks, and Gratitude, with True Holy Love, Namaste, to All who Helped in this Clearing and Healing."

NAME OF PERSON   **OPERATOR**   **DATE**

Identity	Value	Hurt	DarkAttached	DarkValues
Hi Aukamura				
Aukamura				
Higher Self				
Soul Group				

Number of Souls in Healee   Values of Souls

Number of Past Lives causing problems - Higher Self: Soul Group   Soul

Values of Past Lives causing problems - Higher Self: Soul Group   Soul

Implanted Devices/Objects: Booby Traps: Life Mission: Forgiveness :

Assemblage Beam: Straight: Centered: Correct Angle:

Energy Suckers: People: Vampires:

Condition of Guardian Angel: **Value of Guardian Angel:**

Value of Akashic Record: **Value of Karma:**

Total Number of Super-Consciousnesses in or around the person:
Value of Super-Consciousness belonging to Person
Values of Super-Consciousness intruding in Person
Dark forces attached, etc., to Super-Consciousnesses - number: values:

Total Number of Consciousnesses in or around the person:
Value of Consciousness belonging to Person
Values of Consciousness intruding in Person
Dark forces attached, etc., to Consciousnesses - number: values:

Total Number of Sub-Consciousnesses in or around the person:
Value of Sub-Consciousness belonging to Person
Values of Sub-Consciousness intruding in Person
Dark forces attached, etc., to Sub-Consciousnesses - number: values:
Is the Sub-Consciousness causing hurts, etc. to protect ?   Still needed ?

<u>**NUMERIC KEY:**</u>   - : Negative   + : Positive
0 = Balanced   1 = Good   2 = Fair   3 = Poor   4 = Bad   5 = Severe   6 = Critical
E.g.   -5 = Highly dangerous, will kill with slightest provocation and little reason.
         +5 = Stubborn in thought, unrelenting, unforgiving - the 'Hanging Judge'

Number of Guides, etc. working with Healee: Values:

Is the Heart operating at all times in True Holy Love, Namaste ?

Is the Subconscious willing to work as a Good Servant of the Heart ?

Is the ego willing to work as a Good Servant of the Heart ?

Number of Entities in and around person's home other than Fragments:

Number of inappropriate energies influencing person:

Number of negative programs accumulated during lifetime:

Total Number of Fragments around person & within mind / sub-conscious:

Other Souls   Own Soul   Baby Souls   Extra Terrestrial   Animal   Other

Values of Fragments intruding in Person:

Any Other Non-Beneficial Interference:

Total Other Negative Influences around person & within mind / sub-conscious:

Other Attachments	Thought Forms	Animal	Plant
Hypnotism	Extra Terrestrial	Hexes/Curses	Other

Values of influences intruding in Person

Past Life problems/influences still to be Healed ?   Number: Values:

Apometric Healing Needed ? (If so, this will be done during sleep time)

OTHER METHODS USED:

Energy System:	Vitality	Main Chakras (Colour Therapy - next pages)
Auric Clearing	Healing Ring	Hands-On Healing EFT
Radionics/Organ	Other Universe	Other Dimension Timelines

<u>**NOTES**</u>

TOUCH STONES - FOR VITALITY

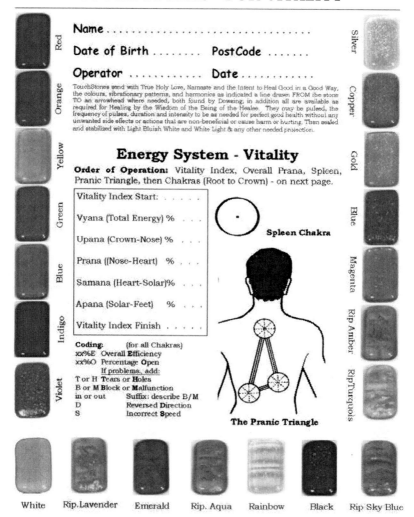

Name . . . .

Date of Birth . . . .   PostCode . . . .

Operator . . . .   Date . . . .

TouchStones send with True Holy Love, Namaste and the Intent to Heal Good in a Good Way, the colours, vibrationary patterns, and harmonics as indicated a line drawn FROM the stone TO an arrowhead where needed, both found by Dowsing, in addition all are available as required for Healing by the Wisdom of the Being of the Healee. They may be pulsed, the frequency of pulses, duration and intensity to be as needed for perfect good health without any unwanted side effects or actions that are non-beneficial or cause harm or hurting. Then sealed and stabilised with Light Bluish White and White Light & any other needed protection.

Energy System - Vitality

Order of Operation: Vitality Index, Overall Prana, Spleen, Pranic Triangle, then Chakras (Root to Crown) - on next page.

Vitality Index Start: . . . . . .

Vyana (Total Energy) % . . . .

Upana (Crown-Nose) % . . . .

Prana ((Nose-Heart) % . . . .

Samana (Heart-Solar)% . . . .

Apana (Solar-Feet) % . . . .

Vitality Index Finish . . . . .

Coding: (for all Chakras)
xx%E Overall Efficiency
xx%O Percentage Open
If problems, add:
T or H Tears or Holes
B or M Block or Malfunction
in or out Suffix: describe B/M
D Reversed Direction
S Incorrect Speed

Spleen Chakra

The Pranic Triangle

Labels (left, top to bottom): Red, Orange, Yellow, Green, Blue, Indigo, Violet

Labels (right, top to bottom): Silver, Copper, Gold, Blue, Magenta, Rip Amber, RipTurquois

Labels (bottom): White, Rip.Lavender, Emerald, Rip. Aqua, Rainbow, Black, Rip Sky Blue

These are printed here in grey-scale - for full colour charts see - www.in2it.ca/HealManual.pdf - FREE Download

Dowse for values using your counting chart and note causes listed under 'coding'.

Use your Pendulum to connect organ and the Touch Stone needed - by swinging between them 'with intent'.

TOUCH STONES - CHAKRAS

Red

Orange

Yellow

Green

Blue

Indigo

Violet

Silver

Copper

Gold

Blue

Magenta

Rip Amber

RipTurquois

Name . . . .

Date of Birth . . . . PostCode . . . .

Operator . . . . Date . . . .

TouchStones send with True Holy Love, Namaste and the Intent to Heal Good in a Good Way, the colours, vibrationary patterns, and harmonics as indicated a line drawn FROM the stone TO an arrowhead where needed, both found by Dowsing; in addition all are available as required for Healing by the Wisdom of the Being of the Healee. They may be pulsed, the frequency of pulses, duration and intensity to be as needed for perfect good health without any unwanted side effects or actions that are non-beneficial or cause harm or hurting. Then sealed and stabilized with Light Bluish White and White Light & any other needed protection.

Top
Back

Top
Front

7

6b   6a

5b   5a

4b   4a

3b   3a

2b   2a

1

Energy System   Main Chakras

White   Rip.Lavender   Emerald   Rip. Aqua   Rainbow   Black   Rip Sky Blue

Continue on this page as on the page for Vitality.

More charts (letter sized, and in full colour) are in the 'Distant Healing manual - a free download from our site.

www.in2it.ca/HealManual.pdf

Character - Attributes & Attitudes

Compared to the average good, fit, and healthy
person of same sex (considered to be 100%)

Self Image:
    Conscious Personality

    Sub-consciousness

Temperament

Emotional Balance

Integrity

Intelligence

Reasoning

Flexibility

Creativity

Good Health

Body Co-ordination

Manual Dexterity

Free of Fear

Free of Worrying

Free of Recreational Drugs,
    Tobacco

        Other

CHARACTERISTIC	HOME	WORK	SOCIAL
Honesty (money, things)			
Truthfulness			
Compatibility			
Dependability			
Loyalty			
Sociability			
Time Keeping			
Problem Solving			
Non-Abuser Violence			
Non-Abuser Verbal			
Non-Abuser Situational			
Non-Abuser Bullying			
Non-Abuser Sexual			

Alcoholic drinks: Non-drinker
Social light drinker   Social medium drinker
Social heavy drinker   Alcoholic /Drunkard

OVERALL ASSESSMENT:

Letter sized forms for Actual Use

You can download the free .pdf file of Chapter 8 which includes the charts and worksheets - then you can select which pages that you want and print them on your printer:

www.in2it.ca/ExorcismWorkLetter.pdf

The Touch Stone pages are in full colour in that .pdf file..

You can download a sample Application Form:

www.in2it.ca/ExorcismApplication.pdf

'HA !' Breathes

At the end of an exorcism I take four deep breathes, exhaling 'HA !' (this is a Huna technique) with the intent to send the energy of these breathes to assist the work being done, whilst I hold my Ptah Pendulum (small coil down, rotating clockwise - to input Love) over the application form and record sheets (in one pile, with the sheet holding the photograph on top).

I do not attempt to control the pitch or tone of the 'HA !' breathes, but have found that my Heart-Mind-Brain team manipulates my vocal chords so that each breath is different, rising in tone above the previous breath.

Generally the time of rotation of my Ptah Pendulum and of the 'HA !' breath coincide - and some times the Pendulum makes slightly different signals, which I believe is movement caused by an Angelic Being.

Notes:

Forgiveness

If you have anger, jealousy, envy, hatred, resentment or seek revenge the you have given a part of your Spirit Consciousness the task of taking such action.

This part is now not able to operate in peace, harmony and love with the rest of your Spirit Consciousness and is probably going to attempt to hurt whoever is involved in this negative emotion.

Due to the law of attraction, it will bring similar fragments to you - and it is likely that you will be hurt, perhaps by attracting illness and disease associated with such emotional thoughts and feelings.

It is most important that you take all needed action to eradicate such thoughts, and so bring back any parts of your Spirit Consciousness so that all parts are again working together in peace, harmony, and love - preventing any potential fragmentation.

You need to forgive all who have ever caused you problems, ask forgiveness from all who you have thought of hurting, and also to forgive yourself - perhaps the hardest part of all!

It is most important that you successfully and completely forgive all who have ever caused you hurt or harm, forgiving from Soul and Spirit as well as mind.

This can be very difficult, especially in cases of abuse (or worse) by family members or those you trusted.

It is suggested that in such cases you accept that what was done occurred as a result of karma (or possession), and was not directly the fault of the perpetrators.

The key is to find some 'reason' to allow you to forgive, no matter how difficult this is for the rational mind. Failure to be so forgiving will prevent any exorcism from being effective - you may get short term relief, but problems will re-occur.

The following statement is to be considered carefully.

If acceptable, ask your "Wisdom of my Being, the Wisdom of my Body, my Heart, my sub-conscious, and all that are involved in any way, to align with Pure Heart and be correctly grounded, to accept and implement this intention with True Holy Love, Namaste, to be effective in all my life at all times and in all circumstances" and then read it aloud three times to make it fully effective. You must be honest and sincere!

"I [name], with True Holy Love, Namaste, do hereby forgive all who have caused hurts, harm, problems, and emotional, mental, and spiritual traumas to me and to all or any in my families, communities, and associations. I forgive you completely in all ways and in all aspects, in all planes of existence, in all domains, and in all dimensions. Whatever has been caused is now in the past and is of no importance to me now and does not matter to me any more. I am now free of all such causes and their effects."

"I [name] do humbly and sincerely apologize for all the hurts, harm, problems, and emotional, mental, and spiritual traumas that I have caused to all life forms, including all that were knowingly or unknowingly, intentionally or unintentionally caused, in all my life including all past lives of myself and all in my Soul families."

"I [name] do humbly and sincerely ask forgiveness for all the hurts, harm, problems, and emotional, mental, and spiritual traumas that I have caused to all life forms, including all that were knowingly or unknowingly, intentionally or unintentionally caused, in all my life including all past lives of myself and all in my Soul families."

"I [name] do humbly and sincerely ask Angelic help to Heal, clear, and remove from my total Being all emotional triggers attached or linked to my cellular, aural, and other memories of all these hurts, harm, problems, and traumas, and to keep me so free of non-beneficial emotional triggers in all nows and at all times."

"I [name], with True Holy Love, Namaste, do hereby bring back to me all Energies and Soul parts that have left me or been lost in any way, and do humbly and sincerely ask Angelic help to Heal them with Unconditional True Holy Love, Namaste, so that they can be in their rightful place".

"I [name], with True Holy Love, Namaste, do hereby release all non-beneficial Energies and Soul parts that have come to me in any way and for any reason, and do humbly and sincerely ask Angelic help to Heal them with Unconditional True Holy Love, Namaste, and take them to be in their rightful place".

"I [name] do humbly and sincerely send my Love, Gratitude, and Thanks with True Holy Love, Namaste, to all who so help and assist me in this forgiveness."

Notes

Entity Healing and Protection

It is understood that 'All That Is' (and all that 'Is Not') is the result of Tiny Baby Cosmic Energies doing different dances at different speeds in various planes of existence to form separate Beings who have different jobs.

The simplest dance teams could be called Lights, then Tinys and Smalls; perhaps these correspond to photons, electrons, sub-atomic particles - and so on.

Every Tiny Baby Cosmic Energy (and most of their simplest dance teams) Love, Feel, Think, and Act - they are Beings in their own right, and most want to have a good life helping others.

When they join a higher level team their energy, etc., is used by the leader of the team to do the job of the team; in some cases the leaders have been hurt, been given bad jobs to cause hurts, or are bosses who like to hurt others.

I am writing a book 'Elemental Creation' which goes into far more detail - but for our purpose here accept that there are healers in the 'True Holy Love Namaste' team who can dismantle such teams and will heal all who have been hurt.

This is similar to removing the bad high command of an army and assigning the soldiers to a different army - the 'Force for Good'.

The following procedures can be used to heal any entity (or group) that is attacking you - or other people.

They are even more powerful when done with a Pendulum to magnify their effects.

Simple Attack

If a person feels that they are under attack, a simple response is to locate and (if possible) identify the attacker.

This can be done by placing your awareness where the attack is felt, and then asking questions such as "If I knew The identity of the attacker, what would the correct answer be?"

Then speak in your mind to the attacker:
"I love you, all associated with you, and all that is in you all unconditionally, and send you Ho'oponopono with good God energy, Blessing 995 and 885, and Healing 997 and 887, all with this wonderful dream Namaste and True Holy Love Namaste itself; I send these to you extra, extra pure, extra, extra special, and extra, extra strong."

Severe Attack
I open with my Heart
In True Holy Love, Namaste
And that Love of Truth.

I send True Holy Love, Namaste
To the entity (*describe it by its actions*)
And to All Associated with you
And to All that are in each of you
Including All the Tiny Baby Cosmic Energies, Elementals,
And all their Families and Teams
I give you unconditional love.

I tell each and every one of you that I Love you more than I love myself.
But I do not like Bad Behaviour.

I send you all True Holy Love, Namaste
With Ho'oponopono.
With Good God Energy.
With Blessing 995 and 885 to help you in your path of life.
With Healing 997 and 887 including all Dances, Vibrational Patterns, Energies, Essences, Frequencies, and Fragrances that Heal Good in a Good Way with True Holy Love, Namaste.
With Ultra High Energy Howls and Lasers of Violet Light to Smash all defences against the Force for Good.
With Ultimate Light Dissolvers of All Negativity.
With the Wonderful Dream Namaste.
And with True Holy Love, Namaste itself.

I send these to all of you
Extra Extra Extra Extra Extra Extra Special
Extra Extra Extra Extra Extra Extra Pure
Extra Extra Extra Extra Extra Extra Strong

I send all this to you three times more
And three times more I send it to you all
And three times more I send to each and every one of you
True Holy Love, Namaste
With Ho'oponopono.
With Good God Energy.
With Blessing 995 and 885
With Healing 997 and 887
With Ultra High Energy Howls and Lasers of Violet Light to
Smash all defences against the Force for Good.
With Ultimate Light Dissolvers of All Negativity.
With the Wonderful Dream Namaste.
And with True Holy Love, Namaste itself.

I tell each and every one of you that I Love you more than I
love myself.
But I do not like Bad Behaviour.
I Ask each and every one of you
Do you Like to Hurt Others
Or Love to have a Good Life?
I Tell each and every one of you
Judge Yourselves NOW!

In our wonderful team Namaste
I / We place all our Trust.

Go now to be Healed with True Holy Love, Namaste, in
whatever way is best for All Creation.

*The result is that the energy / force of the bad entity is
taken away - and that of the Force for Good is increased.
This happens because the Tiny Baby Cosmic Energies (and
their families and teams) have 'changed sides'.
The Bad Controllers are now easily Healed in a similar
way.*

Clearing your Energy Field

You are responsible for maintaining your own energy field - this useful statement can help:

"I translate, transmute, transform, transfigure, release and repair all original causes, core beliefs and effects related to (*fill in the blank with what you want to clear*) replacing these with unconditional love; I do so throughout all time space and dimensional matrices both known or unknown. I declare it so and so it is. Thank you. I establish that my trigger point is my third eye. Whenever I touch my finger to my third eye I undertake and complete a deep clearing. I declare it is so. It is done. Thank you."

Deep Clearing

The 'deep clearing' is available at Tyhson Banighen's site:

http://energydetective.ca/2012/dowsing-2/deep-pendulum-clearing/

Books published by the Holistic Intuition Society

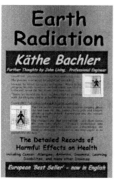

Earth Radiation

The classic record of Käthe Bachler's research into noxious energies involving 11,000 people in more than 3,000 homes and work places in 14 countries. 'Further Thoughts' by John Living.

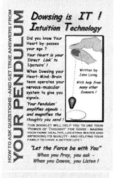

Sleep Well, Be Healthy

A concise summary based on 'Earth Radiation' designed as a booklet for distribution by Dowsers and Health Professionals aware of such noxious energies. Bulk orders for booklets, or buy the E-Book first to have a look at it.

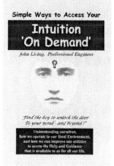

Your Pendulum

Booklet with a glass bead Pendulum - designed as an 'Xmas stocking stuffer' to help people to learn about Dowsing - and how Dowsing can help them (and others). Excellent concise instructions. Bulk orders for booklets, or buy the E-Book first to have a look at it.

Intuition 'On Demand'

We all have Intuition - but many have problems getting help when needed. This book explains how you can do just that ! This book is 'entry level' - for people who are not experts !

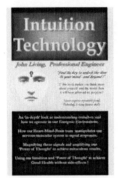

Intuition Technology

Dowsing is 'IT' - an in-depth look at understanding ourselves and our environment, full instructions on improving our Dowsing abilities, and advanced knowledge about our total energy bodies and how we can work with the energies to improve health.
This book includes almost all of "Intuition On Demand" !

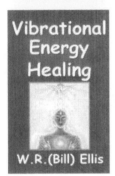

W.R.(Bill) Ellis

Vibrational Energy Healing

By the recognized Master Healer Bill Ellis - who gives hints for using a Pendulum for Healing, explains improvements made by Bill to many Healing modalities, and introduces some completely new methods of Healing - both for using 'Hands On' procedures and for distant Healing.   John Living edited this book.

Books to be published in 2013

Holistic Healing with Heart

"We are all the same" - so can communicate for Healing on a 'Heart to Heart' basis, including changing the vibrational patterns that cause illness. Using Clones to help, working with the Angelic Beings, accessing improved conditions in all time and space, including other dimensions.

Elemental Creation

An unusual look at how the various planes developed, how they interface in the physical and other dimensions, and how human beings can influence all of creation.

NOTE: Sleep Well, Be Healthy and Your Pendulum
Bulk orders of these 2 booklets are available from the Holistic Intuition Society.
The other books can be purchased on Amazon or from the Holistic Intuition Society - note that our prices include shipping and handling worldwide.

Lightning Source UK Ltd.
Milton Keynes UK
UKOW02f2027190616

276649UK00002B/10/P